BODY 4 GOLF:

GETTING INTO THE SWING

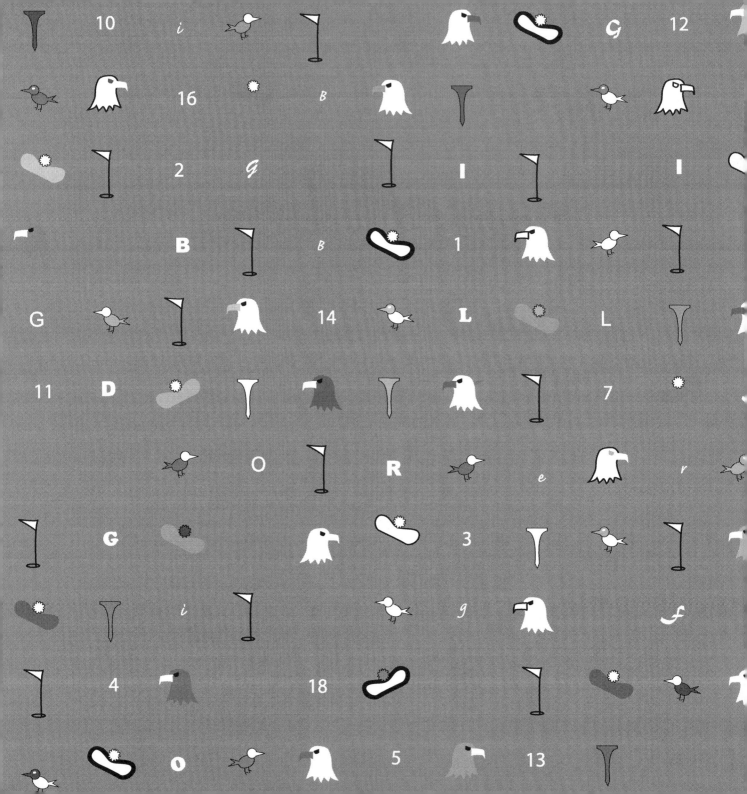

BODY 4 GOLF:

GETTING INTO THE SWING

Dawn Lipori, M.S.P.T.

Diva Dog Publishing, Inc.
P.O. Box 1819
Windermere, Florida 34786
www.divadogpublishing.com

Illustrator: Cheryl Lipori www.liporidesign.com (except where noted otherwise.)
Editor: Brooks Nohlgren www.booksbybrookes.com
Designer: Nicole Recchia www.nicoledesign.net
Shannon Littrell Photography www.shannonlittrell.com

This book does not diagnose medical problems or suggest treatment. Please consult with your physician before beginning any new exercise program.

DEDICATION

This book is dedicated to my loving friends and my faithful dog Tess.

To Lee and Beverly Janzen who had the faith to refer me to all their family, friends, and colleagues. To Carl Rabito who taught me the golf swing and asked me many insightful questions that formed the basis of this book. To Dr. Loren Rex, D.O., better known as Bear, who taught me about the body, how to teach myself, and how to learn from every client. And of course, to all the golfers both professional and recreational who allowed me to learn from their bodies, and develop my theories working with them.

This book would not have been possible without help from many wonderful friends and expert professionals. My friends and colleagues Bob Cohen and Jon Laking who took time from their busy lives to advise me on the biomechanical content of the book. Thanks also to Nathan Lundiski, my model, and to Claudia Lucas, my model photographer, and also to Cheryl Lipori, my amazing and talented sister who painstakingly drew every illustration. Further gratitude to Shira McKinley, my good friend, who helped with legal contracts and unflagging support, and to Kay Robinson, my intuitive business coach, who helped me personally, professionally, and spiritually. With Kay's help, I uncovered my personal strength. I'm also grateful to Wendy Newman, my branding coach, who guided me to my greatest potential and introduced me to some beautiful professionals that became part of my professional support team. Much appreciation is also owed to Brookes Nohlgren, my editor, who helped to turn my information and experience into the book you are holding. Thank you to Nicole Recchia, my book designer, who brought the book to life, to Chip Koehlke, my golf content advisor, to Justin Blazer, the handsome golf instructor on the cover, to David Graham, who was brave enough to lay on the ground in front of Justin to photograph him while he drove golf balls. Also thanks to Shannon Littrell who took my personal photo. And finally, big thanks of course, to my personal support team: Tammi, Fern, Karen, Galen, Christina, Julie, Shira, Richard, Galen, Kay, Wendy, Joann, John, Tess, and God.

Body 4 Golf **Table of Contents**

Body 4 Golf **Table of Contents**

We all want an optimal golf swing. Unfortunately, a lack of time, money, proper instruction, and body motion, not to mention the presence of injuries, too often keep us from attaining this elusive goal. And while there are two main areas that can be the cause of a less-than-ideal swing—technical issues (swing dynamics) and flexibility problems (body range of motion or ROM)—just pick up any golf magazine or book and you will see that the focus tends to be put solely on the former issue, overlooking the body's own limitations almost entirely. Up until now, the science of golf swing diagnostics research has centered on using expensive equipment to determine "perfect" angles and "perfect" body positioning relative to the club and the swing path. When the angles are incorrect, the golfer is shown what he or she is doing wrong and asked to correct the problems.

But what if you can't correct these problems? What if your body, despite your effort, determination, focus, practice, and drive, is not capable of moving that way? Your sub-optimal swing pattern is much more likely the result of compensations in one area of your body for a restriction in another, a restriction you are possibly not even aware of. So, though little attention is given to flexibility problems in golf, I have found in my many years of working with top golf athletes that this truly is the bigger, more relevant issue inhibiting the golf swing. Additionally, this often overlooked part of the equation must be fixed *first* before you can address technique. All the expensive equipment, swing aids, and technical advances in the world will not help you if it is your body that is limiting your performance. This is actually very good news, because even small adjustments can make major improvements in your game.

For our bodies to perform at their best, all parts need to move the way they were designed to. This, above all, gives us the best chance at achieving peak performance. If you're like nearly every other of the world's 61 million golfers, it is likely that your body is not moving ideally in every way. That's why I have written this book for you.

Using *Body 4 Golf: Getting into the Swing*, you will discover which body areas you need to improve, perform simple exercises, and then watch your scores get better. My goal is to put your golf game back in your hands, knowing that with the right tools and information you absolutely have the power to improve your game. With this book you can become your own body expert, truly turning it into a body for golf. After following the recommendations of the book, not only will your performance improve, but your chances of injury will also decrease, giving you the opportunity to golf well into your golden years.

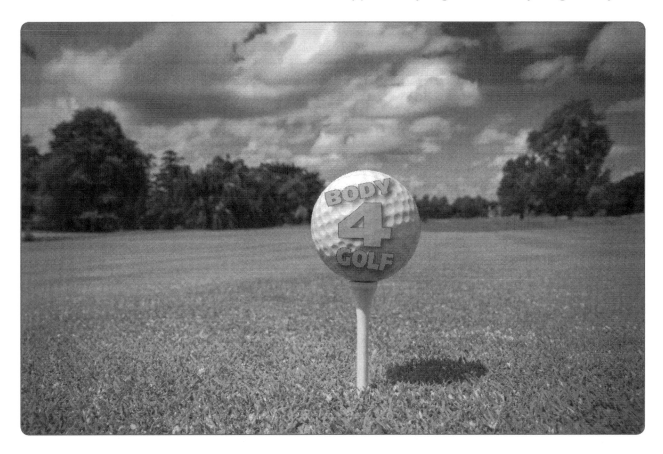

This book was designed to help you distinguish between the two main causes of a sub-optimal golf swing: flexibility problems (your body does not move that way) and technical issues (you need golf swing training or practice). To accomplish this, it discusses body mechanics and the golf swing from the body's point of view.

Having worked with over one hundred professional golfers and several hundred recreational golfers over nearly two decades, I recognize that there are differences in body types as well as swing styles, and that results will vary between individuals. I believe that the perfect swing is the one that works best for you. A small change in range of motion (ROM), say half an inch, could be all you need to succeed with the golf swing you desire.

This book was written as if you where a right-hand golfer. Please reverse "rights" and "lefts" if you are a left-hand golfer. This book also assumes that you are a practicing golfer, familiar with the five phases of the golf swing: address, backswing, downswing, impact, and follow-through.

Enjoy learning about your body and improving your swing!

Forward by Lee Janzen

I have been fortunate enough to play on the PGA tour for over 20 years. There are many factors that have been a part of being able to compete for a long time. I have needed to change over the years to keep up with the advancements in many areas of the game of golf.

When I first started I didn't know much about the equipment I used, but I have learned a lot about what works best for me and why.

Hardly anyone was working out on tour in 1990. Then players got into physical fitness, and how to work out continued to evolve. Just going to the gym and lifting weights and doing cardio was the beginning. Now most players have trainers that are not only putting programs in place, but golf specific training.

Even though we have a pretty good idea which muscles are most important for golf, it's not enough. Building stronger golf muscles won't help you if you are lacking mobility and stability throughout your body.

I have known Dawn Lipori for over 10 years. She has shown me exercises that have been helpful and I trust her knowledge of the human body.

I hope you read this book carefully and find out where you can improve your golf game. Have you ever considered why you or someone else just couldn't seem to make that big hip turn? Maybe it wasn't your swing, but you lacked the proper mobility in your ankles or hips or somewhere else. I think you will be excited about the chance to get better by doing some new exercises.

Thanks for picking up *Body 4 Golf* and enjoy!

Lee Janzen
U.S. Men's Open Champion, '93, '98

Praise for
BODY 4 GOLF: GETTING INTO THE SWING

"Body 4 golf will dramatically improve your flexibly and range of motion for golf quickly. "

Chip Koehlke, PGA
— Director of Instruction, Chip Koehlke Golf Academy

"Thirty years ago, when I first took up golf as a teenager in a Hawaii Junior Golf Program, I remember hitting thousands of golf balls at the driving range day after day, and playing 36 holes of golf carrying my own bag in the blistering heat and humidity with no problem. I was taught more by "feel" than by technique and over the years, continued to play competitive golf.

With two young children and working as a full-time small animal veterinarian, it is now a luxury to play a round of golf. I have become a recreational golfer and my body has lost a great deal of strength and flexibility over the years. My drives are not as long off the tee, I am not able to make as big a turn on my backswing, certain parts of my body ache after playing that never did before, and it takes longer for my body to recover after playing a round.

After reading Body 4 Golf, I performed each test in the book and saw where my weaknesses were. Dawn's tests were easy to understand and follow. Doing some of the exercises before playing a round significantly helped my range of motion and flexibility while playing and minimized the discomfort the day after the round.

I think any golfer…beginner, competitive, professional or recreational, can learn a great deal from this book. It may save you an unnecessary trip to a physician, physical therapist, or massage therapist. It is easy to read, the tests are easy to execute, and it is easy to refer to when you want to learn more about your body. Every golfer and every swing coach needs to read this book and incorporate this into their golf program.

Thank you, Dawn, for allowing me to learn from your years of wisdom and dedication to the sport of golf. I hope to be playing into my golden years."

Dr. Kim Carvalho, Dipl. ABVP

"I have spent the last 36 years in professional baseball with the Chicago White Sox in many capacities from player, to coach, to scout, to executive. I have seen what it takes to succeed in a sport both physically and mentally. I was amazed when reading this book that it can apply to almost any sport. It is necessary to build strength and flexibility in order to succeed in any athletic endeavor. Dawn covers all of the aspects needed to succeed in golf and improve your game. Many of us who play the game are not in tip-top shape but her simple way of improving yourself physically will definitely help your golf game. I am sure it would help many of our baseball players too!"

Larry Monroe
— Baseball Advisor for the Chicago White Sox

"After you read *Body 4 Golf*, you will understand the mechanics of how your body can hinder some of your golf performance. Once you realize what your area of weakness is and work on it, you will soon feel a great difference in how your body moves and consequently your swing and performance will improve. The golf swing requires a lot of different moves and nothing better than being able to do them without any restriction."

Camilo Benedetti
— Nationwide Tour Player

The goal of golf is to move your body in a dynamic, or continually moving, patterned sequence, so wouldn't it make sense to train your body and muscles in a similarly dynamic way? Yet few golfers do. Few take full advantage of optimizing their swing by preparing to golf using fluid movement. Instead they rely on a static stretch, teaching the muscle to lengthen in a static position. But to train more effectively toward the functional goal of a fluid golf swing, you must teach your muscles to be flexible in a continually moving situation. Thus, by preparing to golf with dynamic movement, the body and muscle learning is closer to the task of golf and can produce great results.

For a basic understanding of how the body moves to create the golf swing, I will discuss the main body areas involved, how they move, and how to prevent injuries to keep your golf game at its best.

How the Body Moves to Create the Golf Swing

A good swing pattern is a beautiful combination of body motions involving flexibility, coordination, and strength of numerous body parts: the feet, ankles, knees, hips, pelvis, trunk, shoulders, elbows, wrists, and hands. To most simply explain how the body coordinates all of these areas to create your swing, I will divide the body into four main sections:

1. Feet/Ankles

2. Hips/Pelvis/Low Back

3. Trunk/Rib cage

4. Upper Extremities (Arms)

The Role of the Feet and Ankles in the Golf Swing

Key to the golf swing, the feet provide ground contact, increasing the stability of the pelvis and thus the body as a whole. The ankles allow the knees to bend forward over the feet and allow the pelvis to shift from right to left and rotate from right to left. The knees respond to the pelvic motion and the fixed feet.

The Role of the Hips/Pelvis/Low Back Complex (HPLB Complex) in the Golf Swing

The HPLB complex stabilizes the body while the club is moving. These areas provide the foundation of the body and therefore the swing. Without this foundation, your core will be weak or non-functioning.

The Role of the Trunk/Rib cage in the Golf Swing

The trunk/rib cage is better known as the core. The core is the generator of the golf swing. The core drives the arms making the core the primary source of speed for the golf club. The core and HPLB complex team up to provide your power for the golf swing, fueling both the downswing (or acceleration of the club) and the backswing (or deceleration of the club).

The Role of the Upper Extremities (Arms) in the Golf Swing

The arms ensure the club face contacts the ball properly. The arms are the secondary source of power for the swing. They can add extra speed from the elbow motion as well as wrist motion if these motions are at the appropriate time to create a double-lever arm. This makes the arms the secondary source of speed.

The Importance of Proper Range of Motion (ROM)

The movement of our joints is measured as range of motion (ROM). While there are medically documented average ROMs for each specific joint of the body, for our purposes here it is easier and more functional to look at ROM for the four main body areas that create the golf swing. The golf swing requires large quantities of movement from all four areas, and without proper ROM, a fluid, effective, injury-free swing would be impossible.

Although it is easier to test ROM by dividing the body into four areas, it is still important that each joint in your body functions properly. Knowing the difference between the quality and quantity of ROM is helpful to properly assess each individual joint.

Quality/Quantity of Motion

Range of motion is not just about quantity, meaning how far a joint can move. An example of quantity of motion would be flexing your arm (bringing the arm forward and up) as high as you can. See Figure 1. How far can you raise it?

Range of motion also depends greatly on the quality of motion. This takes into consideration all the parts that move, not just the obvious change in position of the body part. There are many accessory motions, or involuntary small movements, occurring between joints. These accessory motions, including gliding and rotation, occur to constantly adjust and change the angle of alignment of the joints. This is important because joint surfaces are not perfectly smooth or rounded.

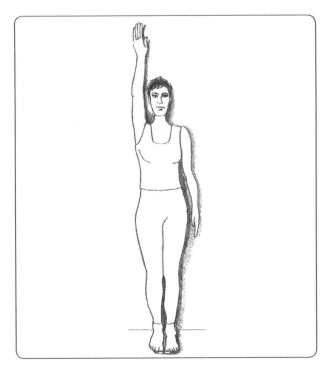

Figure 1

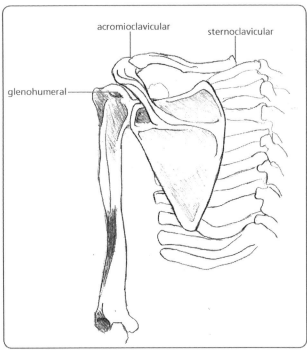

Figure 2

To demonstrate this concept, let's look at an example showing the difference between all the joints involved in the shoulder moving properly (quality) and where it appears that the shoulder has moved well (quantity). Keep in mind that quantity without quality will eventually cause injuries.

The joints directly involved with shoulder motion are the sternoclavicular (breast bone and collarbone), acromioclavicular (shoulder blade and collarbone), and the glenohumeral (shoulder blade and humerus). See Figure 2.

The rib cage, which the scapula (shoulder blade) has to move over, would be indirectly involved. There are also muscles and other tissues that have to lengthen and shorten appropriately to allow the joints to move. If the accessory motions and tissues are efficient, then when you raised (flexed) your arm, the following would occur: the top of the shoulder would have stayed at the same height or slightly elevated, your neck and back would remain in the same position, the scapula (shoulder blade) would have depressed toward the floor and retracted toward the spine, the scapula (shoulder blade) would stay snug to the rib cage, and there would be no bulging of the head of the humerus in the armpit area. See Figures 3 and 4.

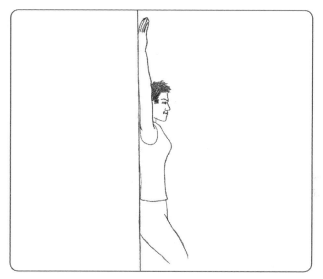

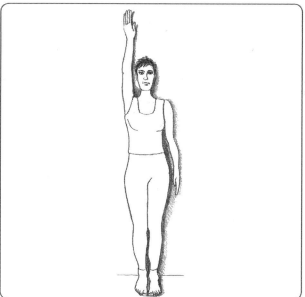

Top, Figure 3   Bottom, Figure 4

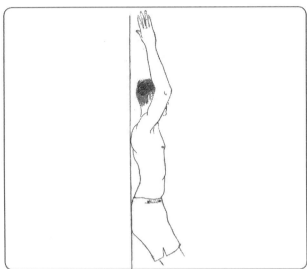

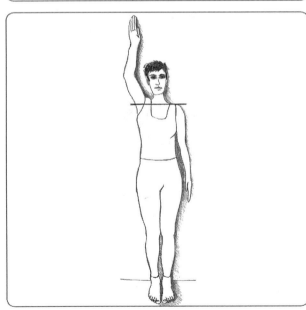

Top, Figure 5   Bottom, Figure 6

If your shoulder rose up, if your spine curves changed, if the scapula hardly moved or winged out from the rib cage, and/or if the humerus bulged in the armpit, then you are compensating for joints that are not moving correctly. See Figures 5 and 6. Compensations over time stress tissues such as bones, cartilage, ligaments, tendons, nerves, muscles, and blood vessels. Over time, compensations cause irritation, inflammation, and eventually pain. Compensations are dysfunctions of body movement.

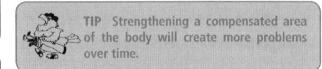

TIP Strengthening a compensated area of the body will create more problems over time.

The Role of Posture

Good posture is absolutely essential to an injury-free golf game. Figures 7 and 8 represent the anatomical alignment of good posture. The medical profession calls this "anatomical neutral." Poor posture such as forward head and rounded back (kyphosis) can limit your swing because you are not starting at neutral. With poor posture, you are beginning with a deficit of ROM.

The posture in Figure 9 presents a severely limited rib cage and will challenge your balance, stability, and rotational ability in all phases of the golf swing. It's easy to see how

Chapter 1: **Body Basics and the Golf Swing**

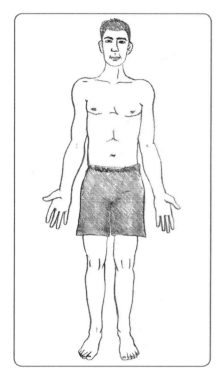
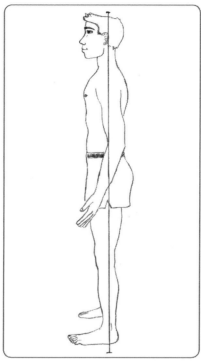
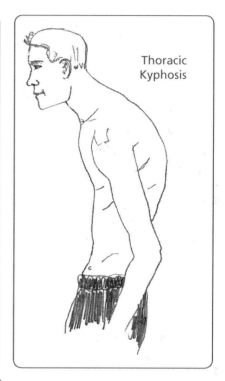

Thoracic Kyphosis

Left, Figure 7   Middle, Figure 8   Right, Figure 9

posture that is poor can severely limit your game. The exercises in this book will help your overall posture as well as your golf swing.

The Importance of Neutral Positioning

With Figure 9, it's easy to see how posture could affect the golf swing. When you are in anatomical neutral position, or good posture, all your joints are in their neutral position. From the neutral position of a joint, the greatest amount of ROM in any one direction is available. Once motion is taken up in one direction, especially if rotation is involved, there is less motion available in the other directions.

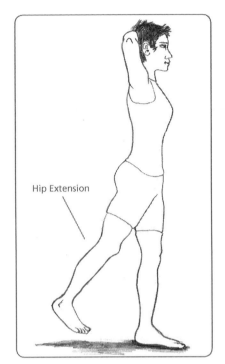
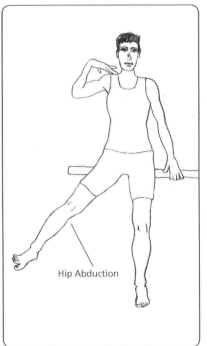
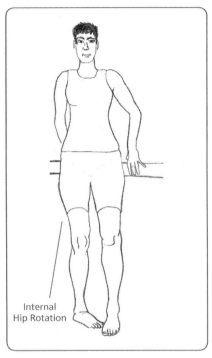

Left, Figure 10   Center, Figure 11   Right, Figure 12

For example, Figures 10, 11, and 12 depict the model fully extending her hip, fully abducting her hip, and fully internally rotating her hip.

Figure 13 combines the motions and depicts the model first fully extending her hip, and from that point fully abducting, and from that point fully internally rotating. Note that there is much less abduction (movement of the leg out to the side away from the body) and internal rotation of the hip (noticed by how far the foot turns in toward the body) with the combined motions.

You can try this for yourself by mirroring the model in the diagrams. Figure 14 represents this same concept in closed position (with the foot touching the ground). This position is similar to the one your right leg is in at or after impact when the right heel is lifted off of the ground. This concept is also very important when deciding stance position at address. How far do you spread your legs past anatomical neutral position?

Chapter 1: **Body Basics and the Golf Swing**

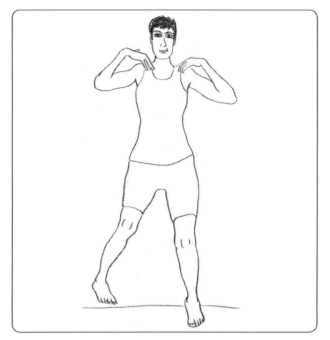

Figure 13

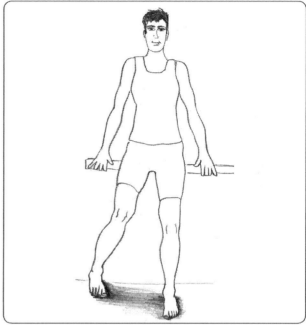

Figure 14

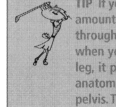

TIP If you are looking for the full available amount of left hip rotation for the follow-through, your stance should be such that when you shift your weight over your left leg, it places the hip in or near to neutral anatomical position, or straight under the pelvis. Then you are ready for full available hip rotation.

Injuries and Other ROM Restrictions

The body is a wonderful machine. It can adapt to multiple areas of dysfunction, compensate by twisting, bending, or overstretching tissues, and still keep you moving. Pain generally occurs when you have exhausted all adaptability of the structural system, or when nothing else can compensate for combined losses of ROM. Keep in mind that you are the sum total of all previous injures after which you did not regain full ROM. This is especially important in golf. In a more adrenaline-based sport like football, you may be able to play with multiple dysfunctions and pain, but the graceful golf swing does not allow such luxury. Body fluidity is essential for a good swing pattern.

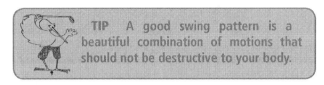
Understanding the path toward dysfunction, or how your body compensates for loss of ROM, and the importance of a solid foundation of good posture will help you recognize when your body is not at peak performance. Using fat shots as an example, you can visibly see how the body absorbs forces resulting in injury and the damaging effect on the golf swing.

Let's say, for example, that you had a particularly rough day on the course and have hit a lot of fat shots. The expression of this impact can be seen in Figure 15. The force travels up the club to the thumb, wrist, radius, interosseous membrane (between the radius and ulna or forearm bones), ulna, elbow, and continues up the chain. The elbow joint, which consists of the ulna, radius, and humerus, is generally where the effects of fat shots are seen. What you initially notice is that your arm does not straighten as well at the elbow. What results is loss of accessory motions (small involuntary movements) between the ulna and humerus, the radius and humerus, and radius and ulna. You continue to golf and, over time, the motion of the swing forcibly asks for extension of the left arm at the elbow. Because your elbow no longer has that motion, the ulna and radius (forearm bones) start to bow.

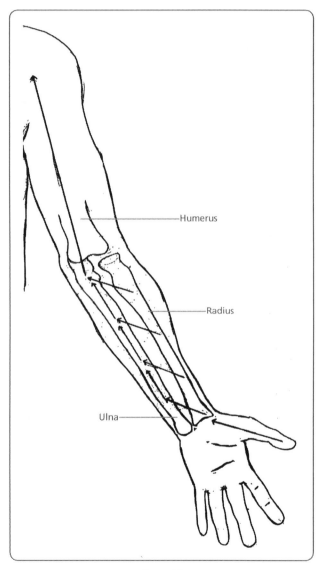

Figure 15

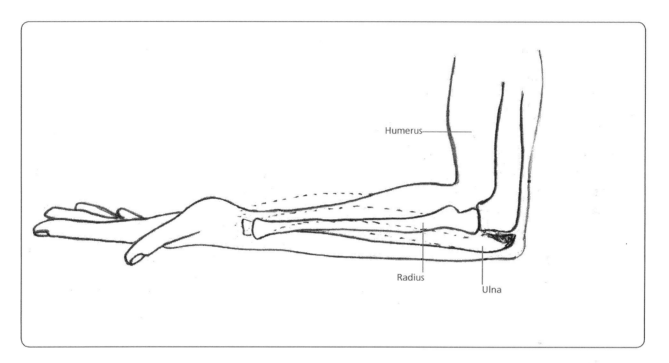

Figure 16

See Figure 16 for an exaggerated example of this. The bones will bow because they are amazingly pliable and will bend and twist before they break. In reality, the very subtle bowing would occur with some separation and twisting of the two bones of the forearm. (The picture shown could not be reproduced by an X-ray because the actual changes are very subtle.) With the bones now sitting bowed, all the muscles are contracting and pulling at improper angles, and you are noticing something is wrong. Because of the bowing, the angles at which the forearm bones attach to the wrist bones are not normal and your wrist and thumb will not move as well. Basically, the impact from the lost ROM in the elbow spreads down to the wrist and hand and up to the shoulder, neck, and ribs. At this point, if asked to straighten your elbow, you appear to have the quantity of full motion. In reality, you are missing quality, because the accessory motions have been compromised. Now think of all your injuries from which you did not regain full ROM, because your body problems are the sum of the dysfunctional areas.

Why Movement Exercises?

A very effective way to regain lost ROM is with movement exercises. Movement exercises take into consideration all the structures of the body and not just the musculature. This type of exercise trains the tissues in a manner similar to how the tissues need to move for the golf swing.

To train the body with dynamic movement, you must have proper alignment and flow. Proper alignment requires that the joints be lined up and held in their neutral positions while performing the exercises. Without proper alignment, the area targeted for improvement may be completely ignored. An example would be trying to improve hamstring flexibility; shifting your hips to the side, away from neutral, changes the angle of pull off of the hamstring muscles. Figures 17 and 18 show proper as well as poor alignment. Generally, if you are not feeling a specific targeted area of tightness, you are probably not aligned correctly. All of the exercises in Chapters 3–6 utilize movement of some kind, allowing flow instead of tightness of tissues and joints, which commonly occurs with static stretching.

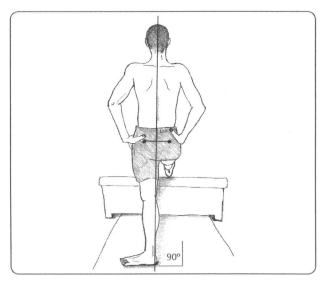

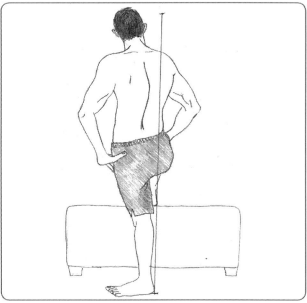

Top, Figure 17   Bottom, Figure 18

Specific alignments are discussed individually in each exercise section.

The Importance of Flow

The golf swing is a beautiful fluid combination of motions, and while it is common to focus on the moving parts as consisting of only joints and musculature, in actuality there are many more tissues and even fluid involved in the body moving to create the golf swing. Flow takes into consideration all the structures of the body, not just the muscles. The basic structures involved are muscles, fascia, nerves, blood vessels, lymph, lymph channels, and organs. The most unfamiliar of these structures may be lymph. Lymph vessels run parallel with the blood vessels. The lymph system acts as a drainage canal network, removing excess fluid from all the body tissues and returning the fluid to the bloodstream.

To illustrate this for you a little bit more, below is an example of motion that involves all the mentioned structures: breathing. As you'll see in the table, this is a lot of moving parts for something we take for granted every day!

All this wonderful movement allows the act of breathing to help you improve motion anywhere in your body. To better understand this, let's take a closer look at the nervous system. All your nerves connect back to the central nervous system (spinal cord, brain, and brain stem).

So if you flex your body down to touch your

Breathing In	Breathing Out
Spinal vertebrae extend	Spinal vertebrae flex returning to neutral
Spinal cord lengthens	Spinal cord returns to resting length
Diaphragm drops down forming a bowl shape	Diaphragm recoils up into its resting shape of an upside down bowl
The liver (from the force of the diaphragm) rotates forward at an oblique angle and drops down toward your feet	The liver moves up toward your head returning to its resting position
The lungs expand by rotating away from the heart up toward your shoulders and down toward the diaphragm	The lungs release air compressing and deflating back to resting position
The ribs elevate	The ribs recoil and depress

hands to the floor, you are asking for flexibility in your entire nervous system. See Figure 19. Now take a breath. As you breathe, the nervous system lengthens and shortens, asking for more motion. Therefore, breathing can be used to improve dynamic nerve flexibility, as well as the flexibility of all other structures involved in breathing. This is a very important concept, as many presumed muscle flexibility problems are actually nerve flexibility problems.

Getting Started

Now that you have a basic understanding of how the body moves to create the golf swing, you are ready to take the next step and test your ROM to see if your body is limiting you.

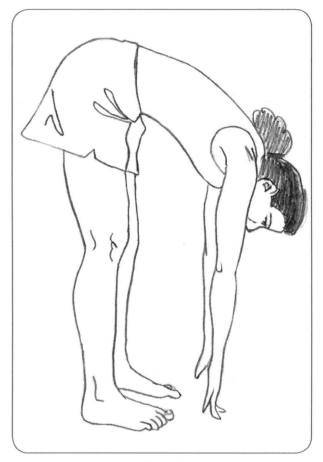

Figure 19

Chapter 2: Self-Testing: How Ready to Swing Is Your Body?

Would you like to know where your body limits your swing and therefore your golf game? This chapter is designed to show you just that. Each test has been meticulously created and/or chosen specifically to address the body motion necessary for golfing. The body has been broken up into four quarters to accomplish this: lower legs, hip/pelvis/low back, trunk/rib cage, and upper extremities (arms). Take the tests, record your results, and then go to the specific chapter for improving each of the four individual body areas.[1]

Most of the tests can be done using a mirror to see your results. Partnering with another golfer and grading each other will work as well. Or, check online at www.body4golf.com to find a certified instructor. Because golf swings and body types differ, there are no exact ranges of motion (ROMs) for each test. Be lenient and grade up if you are undecided between two levels, such as POOR and GOOD. There is a chart in the Appendix A for marking your results. If POOR was your result, consider doing the movement exercises later in the book that correspond to that particular test. If testing results in GOOD or BEST for all four categories, consider doing the Super Seven Warm-Up Exercises in Chapter 9 to maintain fluidity in your swing.

---

1 This book does not diagnose medical problems or suggest treatments. Please consult with your physician before beginning any new exercise program. If at any time during self-testing or exercising you experience pain—other than the resistance of the stretching tissues—consider seeking medical advice. Make sure you read the instructions completely before beginning a test or exercise. Perform exercises and tests slowly, controlling motion. If after two months of diligent exercising your target area does not reap the rewards sought, consider seeking help from a body worker. Go to body4golf.com for a list of manual therapists recommended by the author and other reliable sources.

I also recommend getting to know your body by taking these tests monthly. It is very easy to tune out your body during a busy day or to collect a few minor injuries and not really miss the motion. And though you might be unaware of small losses of motion, they will be apparent in your golf swing. Regularly testing yourself and then improving deficits in ROM will help you attain and/or maintain the swing you desire.

Each test is explained in great detail in its corresponding movement exercise chapter. The movement exercise chapters also contain swing dynamic dysfunctions, the most likely area you will injure if limited in ROM, tips, and movement exercises to improve the corresponding target areas.

Now, let's get started testing for your swing!

Lower Leg Testing

TEST #1: The Three-Way Ankle Test

The Ankle Test has three parts. Part 1 is looking for the motion needed for you to be properly balanced in the stance phase as well as throughout your swing. Parts 2 and 3 are looking for whether your lower leg/ankle/foot complex has the ability to move properly for the follow-through phase of the swing. Testing BEST for all three phases means you should be properly balanced in your stance phase and rotating effectively over your left foot, keeping your right foot contacting the ground as long as possible for the follow-through.

Part 1: Stand with your legs hip-distance apart and your feet flat. Your feet should be facing directly forward. Your feet are aligned, or considered facing forward, when the knee is directly over the second toe. See Figure 20. Your feet should stay flat—touching the floor—at all times during the test.

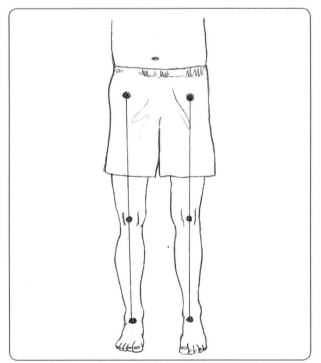

Figure 20

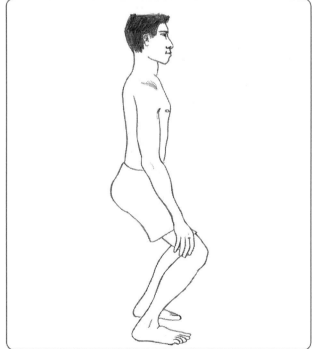

Figure 21

Now bend your knees, letting them come forward over your feet. Do not drop your buttocks as if you were squatting. Instead, keep your upper body and waist upward as you bend. See Figure 21. The test is complete when your ankles stop moving.

To check your results, first look to see if your feet moved. If they moved, you'll need to start over and try again, being sure to keep your feet fixed. There is no need to force the motion. After performing the test properly, look to see where your knees ended. Optimally, you want your knees to be directly over your second toes. See Figure 22.

If your knees look like any of the examples in Figures 23 and 24, then consider doing the exercises in Chapter 3. If your knees fall inside or outside of the second toe, it's very likely that your knees are also naturally falling into this position during the golf swing instead of staying relatively straight.

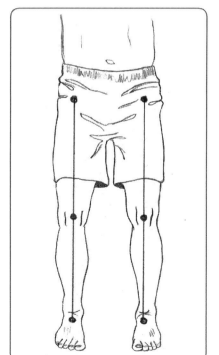 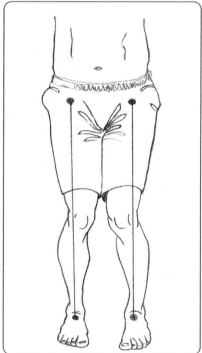 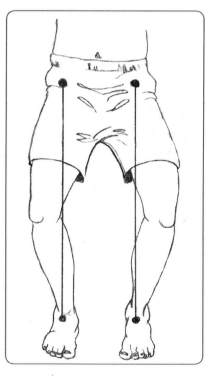

Left, Figure 22   Center, Figure 23   Right, Figure 24

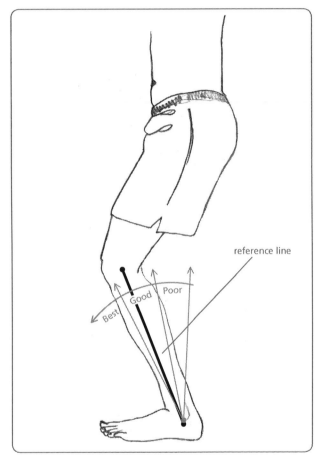

reference line

Best Good Poor

Figure 25

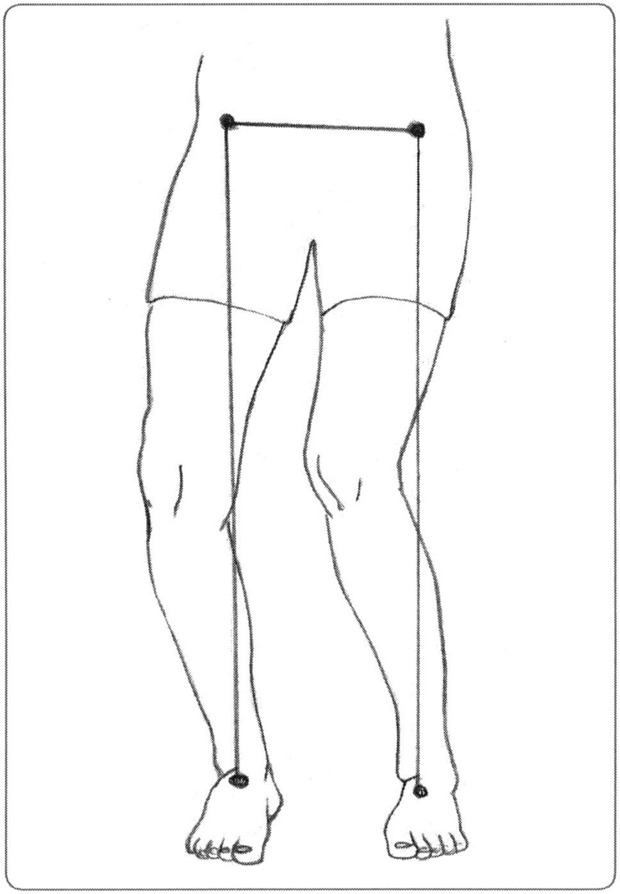

Figure 26

Figure 25 shows POOR, GOOD, and BEST results, for this test, by determining where your reference line falls within the gauge.

Part 2: Begin the test with your legs in the same position as you started Part 1, only this time when you bend your ankles, take both knees an equal distance to the right of center. See Figure 26.

Did your feet stay flat on the floor? If your feet shifted, repeat the test with your feet fixed. Figure 27 shows POOR, GOOD, and BEST

Chapter 2: **Self-Testing: How Ready to Swing is Your Body?**

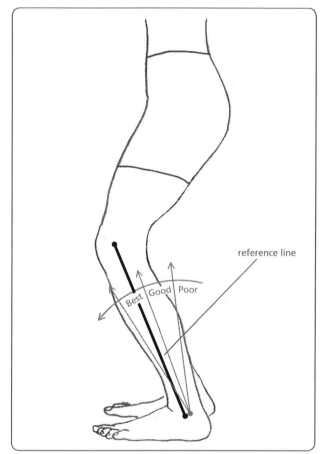

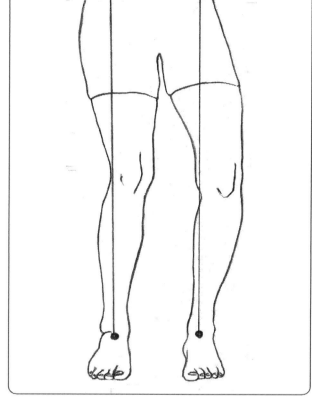

reference line

Best | Good | Poor

Figure 27, Figure 29

Figure 28

results for this test, by determining where your reference line falls within the gauge.

Part 3: Now repeat Part 2, this time taking your knees an equal distance to the left of center. See Figure 28. Did your feet stay flat on the floor? If

your feet moved, repeat the test with the feet fixed. Figure 29 shows POOR, GOOD, and BEST results for this test, by determining where your reference line falls within the gauge.

Hip/Pelvis/Low Back Testing

TEST #2: Hip/Pelvis/Low Back Rotation

The Hip/Pelvis/Low Back Rotation test shows the ability of your pelvis and low back to rotate over your right hip for the backswing and over the left hip for the follow-through. Stand with your feet hip-distance apart, facing straight forward from your body, and with your arms straight out to the side. Your knees should align over your second toes. Keep your feet flat during the entire test. See Figure 30.

Now rotate your pelvis—first to the left as far as you can go, then to the right as far as you can go. See Figures 31 and 32. Figures 33 and 34 shows POOR, GOOD, and BEST results for this test.

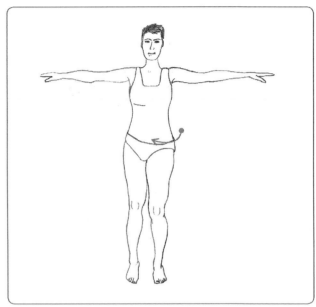

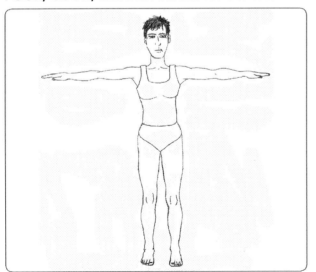

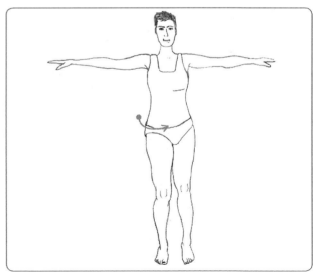

Left, Figure 30   Top Right, Figure 31   Bottom Right, Figure 32

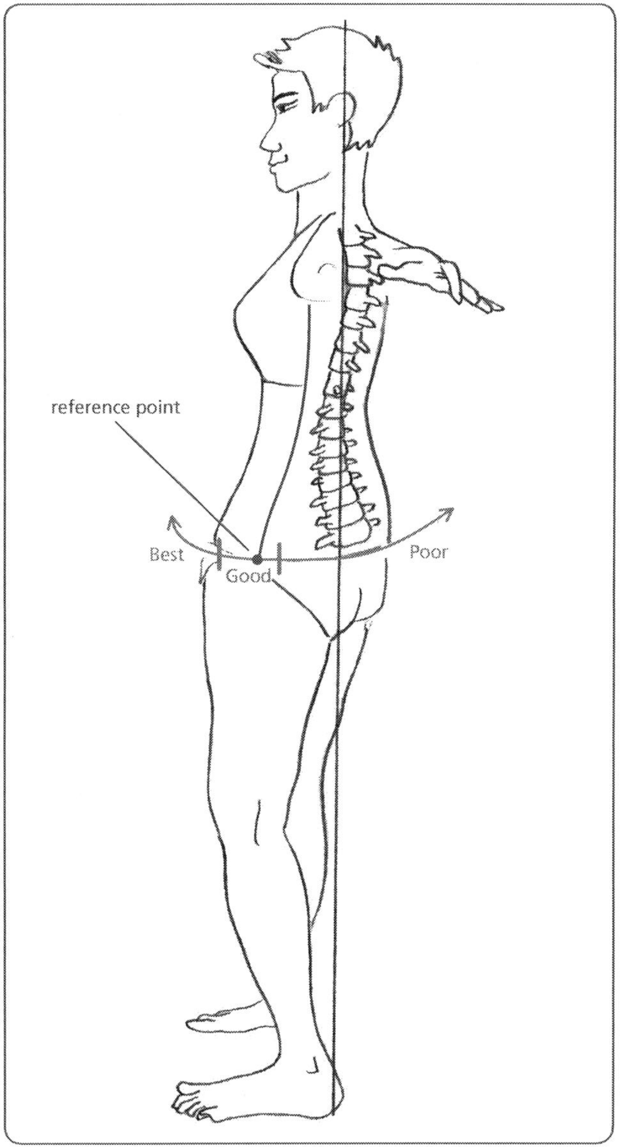

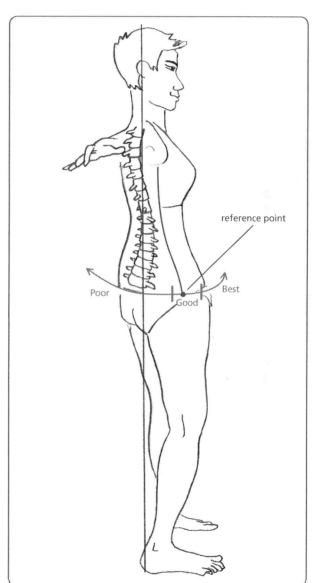

reference point

Best Good Poor

reference point

Poor Good Best

Figure 33

Figure 34

TEST #3: Pelvis Lateral Tilt

The Pelvis Lateral Tilt test shows your body's ability to shift weight left over the left leg and still have enough motion to rotate over both hips for the follow-through. Stand with your left foot on a stair or stool. Make sure your knees are straight and aligned with your legs directly under your pelvis. See Figure 35. To do this, you must hold on to something. Now raise and lower the right side of your pelvis. Your leg should raise and lower with your pelvis. Make sure your pelvis is dropping straight and not rotating forward or backward. See Figures 36 and 37.

For lowering, POOR is 0-1 inch, GOOD is 1-2 inches, and BEST is 2 inches or more. See Figure 38. When raising, POOR is 0-½ inch, GOOD is ½-1 inch, and BEST is 1 inch or more. Repeat with your right leg on the stool, raising and lowering your left leg.

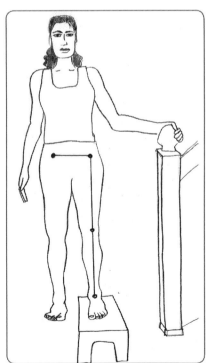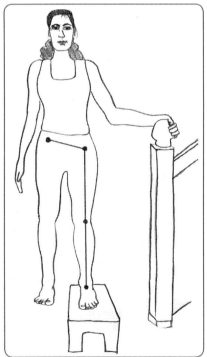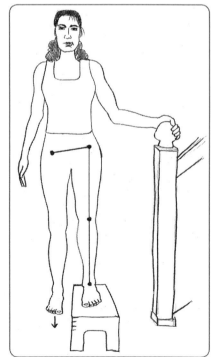

Left, Figure 35   Center, Figure 36   Right, Figure 37

Chapter 2: **Self-Testing: How Ready to Swing is Your Body?**

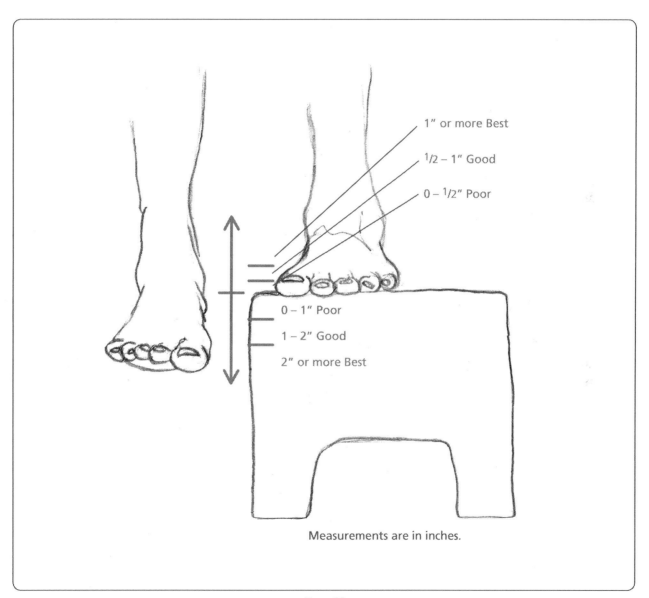

1" or more Best

1/2 – 1" Good

0 – 1/2" Poor

0 – 1" Poor

1 – 2" Good

2" or more Best

Measurements are in inches.

Figure 38

Trunk/Rib cage Testing

TEST #4: Trunk/Rib cage Rotation

This test is looking for the 75-plus degrees of trunk range of motion (ROM) as well as the combined trunk and pelvis motion needed for the swing. Begin by sitting with your feet touching the floor. Bend your trunk forward at the waist as far as you can comfortably go. Your head should be getting closer to the floor. See Figure 39.

Figure 39 shows POOR, GOOD, and BEST results for your ability to bend forward at the waist.

Next, in this position, first rotate right with your arms extended straight from the shoulders, then rotate left. You may need to move your arms around your legs to get into the position of maximum rotation. See Figures 40 and 41. Figures 40 and 41 shows POOR, GOOD, and BEST results for this test. When determining the angle of your rotation, be sure to measure across your shoulders and not from arm to arm.

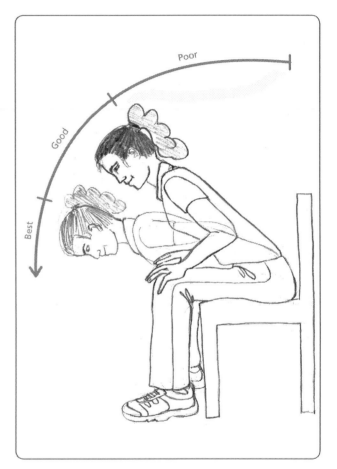

Figure 39

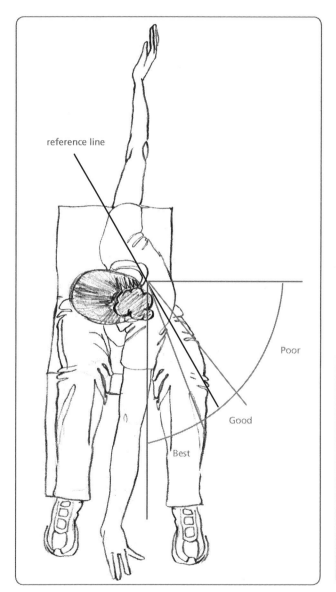

Figure 40

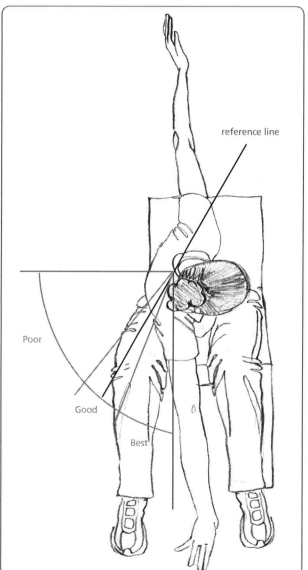

Figure 41

Trunk/Rib cage and Upper Extremity (Arm) Testing

TEST #5: Bilateral Arm Elevation

The Bilateral Arm Elevation Test is checking to see if your trunk mobility restricts your arm motion, which would prevent a full backswing and a proper follow-through.

Stand against a wall with your knees bent, as in Figure 42. Flatten your entire back and rib cage against the wall. If you cannot place your back and rib cage flat, then you have limitations in trunk motion. Next, tuck your chin, straightening your neck. Pull your scapulas (shoulder blades) in toward your spine and down toward the floor, as in Figure 43.

Now raise your arms up over your head toward the wall, allowing only a little change in shoulder height. See Figure 44. BEST would be the entire back flat, with neither shoulder raising up as if you have shrugged them, and arms completely touching the wall. GOOD would be arms close to the wall and small changes in your trunk area, such as not being completely flat. POOR would be any other result. See Figures 44 and 45. Figure 46 depicts back and neck changes that correspond with POOR.

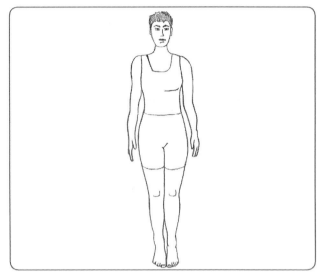

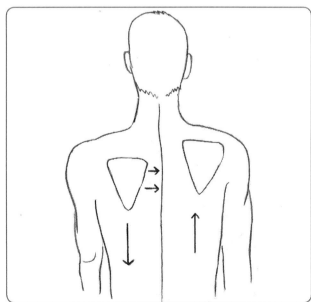

Top, Figure 42   Bottom, Figure 43

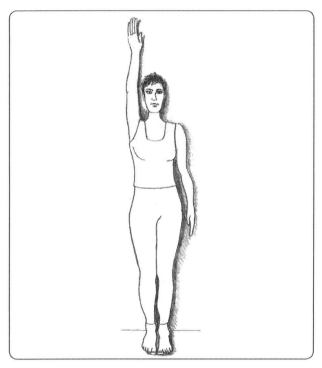

Figure 44

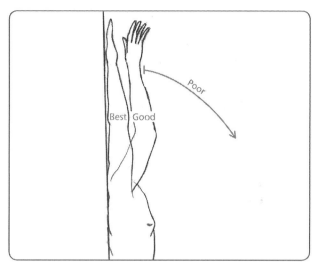

Figure 45

If you scored POOR, either your rib cage is not allowing the motion, the shoulder musculature that attaches to your rib cage is not allowing the motion, and/or your shoulder joints are restricted. If both arms were in the same position, chances are high that the restriction is in the rib cage or core area.

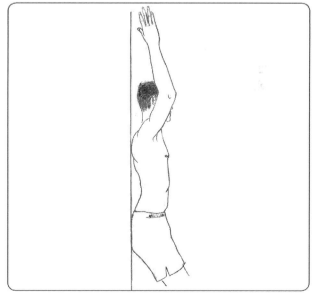

Figure 46

Upper Extremity (Arm) Testing

TEST #6: Shoulder External Rotation

The Shoulder External Rotation Test is looking for the ROM needed in your arms for the backswing and at the end of the follow-through.

Stand with your knees bent with your entire back against a wall. Your feet will be forward from the wall in the position that allows your back to lay flat against the wall. Tuck your chin and straighten your neck. Raise your arms out to the side against the wall to shoulder height. Bend your elbows to 90 degrees. Try to lay your forearms against the wall in this position. See Figure 46. Your back should be flat, your shoulders down, and your scapulas retracted toward the spine. See Figure 47. BEST is pictured. POOR is anything different, including the arching of your back or your head being forward. "Forward head" is when the back of the head does not lay flat or come close to the wall, or when you have to look up toward the ceiling to get the top area of your head to touch the wall behind you.

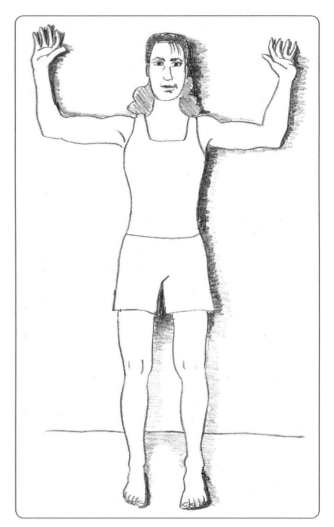

Figure 47

(Turn Page for Test #7)

TEST #7: Prayer Behind Back

This test is checking for the elbow and wrist motion needed for the swing.

WARNING: Perform this test with care! Do not force the position. If you experience pain getting into the testing position, then stop and grade yourself POOR for the test.

Start by sitting, placing your hands palm to palm behind your back in a reverse prayer position, as in Figure 48a. Now roll your hands in toward your spine until they are in a prayer position behind your back. See Figure 48b. Your hands may separate to accomplish this. Move praying hands up your back as much as possible. See Figure 49.

The BEST result is if you can move your hands up your back. GOOD is being able to get into the position. POOR is not being able to get into the position. See Figure 50.

Congratulations! Now that you have completed the self-tests and have some insight into where your range of motion is limiting your golf swing, you may move on to the exercises that will improve your ROM. Chapter 3 has exercises for the feet and ankles, Chapter 4 for the hip/pelvis/lower back, Chapter 5 for the trunk/rib cage area, and Chapter 6 for the upper extremities (arms). If you scored BEST in every self-test, I recommend going to Chapter 7 and using the Super Seven Warm-Up Exercises as a way to keep your swing fluid for the life of your game.

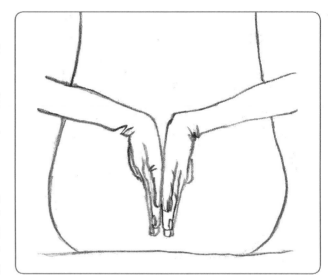

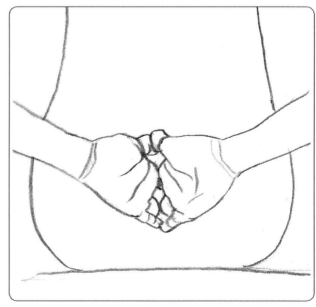

Top, Figure 48a   Bottom, Figure 48b

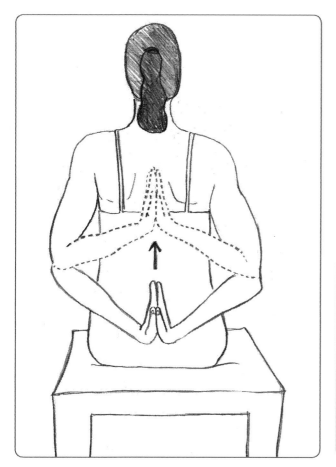

Figure 49

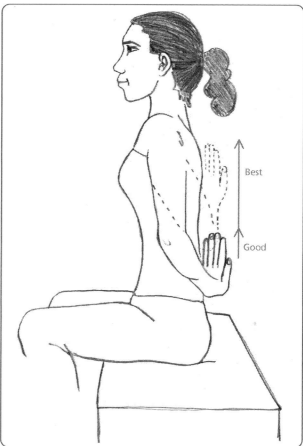

Figure 50

During golf, the feet are positioned for the stance phase and change according to where they end up in the follow-through phase. Other than this, the lower leg/foot/ankle area is not given much thought or attention. After taking the Three-Way Ankle Test in Chapter 2, you may have learned that this area can affect your knee and therefore the entire legs' positioning throughout the golf swing.

In this and the other exercise chapters, you may enjoy learning more about the body mechanics of golf in the Testing/Concepts and Injury sections, or you may want to just skip to the exercises designed to regain any lost motion in this area.

Testing/Concepts

The Three-Way Ankle Test, described in Chapter 2, tests for the lower leg/ankle/foot complex motion needed for all phases of the golf swing. Beginning with the stance phase, if one or both

ankles are restricted, the knees will not move forward over the ankles. Instead, you will have to drop your buttocks lower to the ground and exaggerate your forward bending at the waist to find a balancing position that is not optimal for the golf swing. In this disadvantageous position, the balance and stability needed for the entire swing will be challenged. When you drop your buttocks, you also lose valuable hip/pelvis/low back motion needed for the swing. (Hip/pelvis/low back motion will be discussed in Chapter 4.) This buttocks-dropping position also taxes the calves, quadriceps, hip flexors, and low back musculature. These muscles will be working very hard to keep you from falling over, leaving less power for your golf swing. During the follow-through phase, there is rotation occurring between each lower leg and the corresponding ankle. If the right ankle is restricted, the right heel can be lifted off the ground to compensate. Optimally, the right foot should remain in contact with the ground as long as possible to allow the trunk and pelvic musculature every advantage to decelerate the club properly.

 TIP Decelerating the club in a controlled manner is important for preventing injuries.

If the left ankle is restricted, the left foot can be placed with the toe out to the left in the stance phase. This position is generated from the left hip rotating out from the body or externally rotating. The left leg can be externally rotated beginning from the stance phase, to compensate for loss of ankle ROM. This externally rotated position changes how the hip and pelvic musculature function.

If the restricted left ankle is placed straight, then the knee will have to externally rotate more to compensate. The knee was not designed to rotate that much and will stretch the soft tissues and begin to break down. Over time, this hypermobility (more mobility then what is considered normal) at the knee may cause internal derangement (meniscus tears) and/or strained collateral ligaments (ligaments on the sides of the knees). If your left knee is restricted and cannot compensate by becoming hyper mobile, then you will present with limited pelvic rotation and will probably side bend your trunk to compensate.

Injuries
This section combines normal results from biomechanical (joint motion) breakdown as well as observations I have made over the years in my clinic.

A wide variety of problems may occur from restricted ankles. The most common areas of dysfunction resulting from this restriction tend to be the lumbar (low back) musculature, lumbar vertebrae, lumbar vertebral discs, knees, and feet. Generally, knee problems such as anterior positioned tibia, strained medial collateral ligament, and patella tracking problems manifest at the onset of the injury, called the acute phase. In such cases, pain would be felt in the front of the knee joint, medial (inside of the leg) knee joint, and under or around the patella (knee cap). The acute phase occurs soon after loss of ROM of the ankles. Low back pain and foot pain generally occur after long periods of walking on restricted ankles. Non-traumatic anterior cruciate ligament (a major ligament in your knee) tears often result from a restricted ankle below it.

 TIP Injuries result in areas above and below restricted area.

If you tested POOR or would like to improve your GOOD rating for the ankle test, consider doing the movement exercises listed that follow.

Exercises

Three-Way Ankle

Setup is just like the test. Start by taking your knees forward, then equally to the right, then forward again, and then equally to the left. Repeat 4–12 times. There is no need to force motion at the end range, just keep moving. See Figure 51.

Calf Lengthening

This flexibility exercise can be done using a stair or a wall. Make sure you have something you can hold on to. Start with the left leg straight, bringing it forward from the hip while placing your foot against the wall. Position your left foot with toes angled up toward your head. See Figure 52. Your right leg should be slightly behind you. Your left toes should be making contact with the step or wall. You should be aligned as follows: your right foot should be level and pointing straight ahead, your right knee and patella (knee cap) should be facing forward and in line with your second toe, and your pelvis should be level vertically and not rotated. See Figure 53.

If you are having trouble aligning, back up from the wall or stair and give your foot and

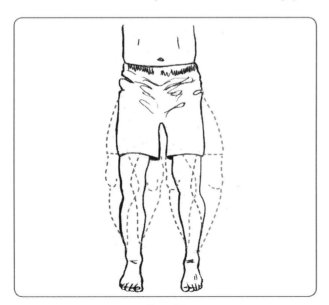

Figure 51

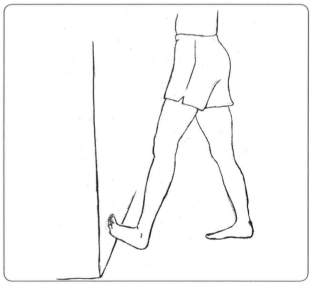

Figure 52

Chapter 3: **Exercises for the Feet and Ankles**

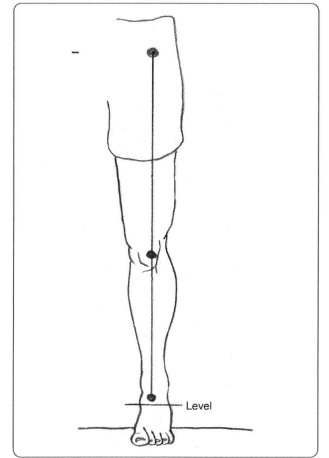

Figure 53

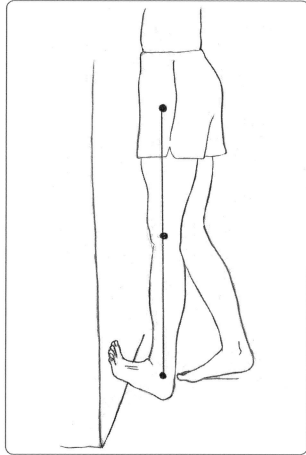

Figure 54

ankle more room. Now start the motion by bending at the left ankle, bringing your whole body forward as a unit. To do this, come up on the right leg's toes. See Figure 54. Move forward until you feel resistance and then lower back to the starting position. Resistance should be felt anywhere in the calf (back part of the lower leg) or ankle area. Complete 4–12 repetitions and then switch your legs to work the right calf.

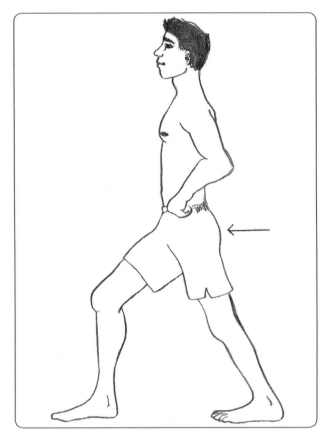

Figure 55

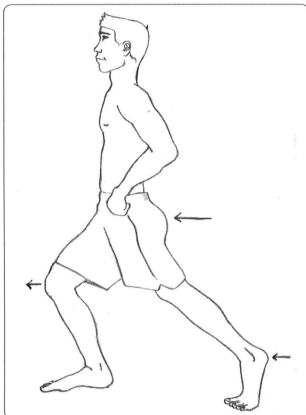

Figure 56

Plantar Lengthening

"Plantar" refers to the bottom of your foot. Lean your whole body forward over your foot, keeping the left leg in front of you. Position yourself with slight resistance to more ankle motion. See Figure 55. Keep your pelvis level and not rotated. Move forward, bending the knee of the left leg and coming up on your toes as your body continues to progress forward. See Figure 56. Continue until you feel resistance, and then come back to the starting position. Resistance should be felt on the bottom of your foot or the ankle area. Complete 4–12 repetitions and then switch to work the left foot.

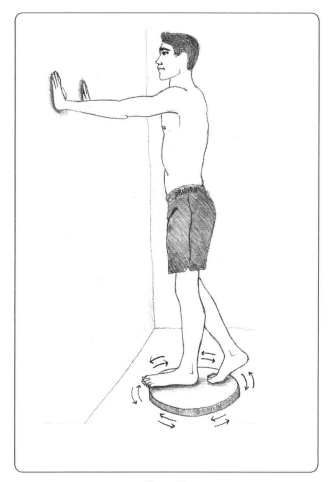

Figure 57

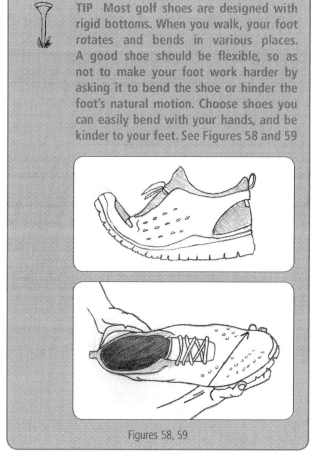

See Figures 58 and 59

Figures 58, 59

Small Circle Balance Board

Place your foot on the board[2] such that the inside and outside bumps of the ankle (the maleoli of the tibia and fibula) are aligned with the middle of the balance board. Place the board on a nonskid surface where you can hold on to something for balance. Move just your foot and ankle in a circle trying to get each edge of the board to contact the floor. Repeat 4–12 revolutions per foot both clockwise and counter-clockwise. See Figure 57.

TIP Most golf shoes are designed with rigid bottoms. When you walk, your foot rotates and bends in various places. A good shoe should be flexible, so as not to make your foot work harder by asking it to bend the shoe or hinder the foot's natural motion. Choose shoes you can easily bend with your hands, and be kinder to your feet. See Figures 58 and 59

TIP There is often a direct correlation between loss of ankle motion and low back pain.

Feet Sitting

For this exercise, begin on the floor as in Figures 60, 61, and 62, placing your feet with toes fully pointed. Your thighs should be directly over your calves. Make sure your legs are hip-distance apart. Now move your buttocks down toward your legs until you feel a slight resistance in the thigh or ankle area, and then lift up 1–2 inches. At first you may not approximate buttocks to feet as depicted in Figures 60–63. Repeat 4–12 repetitions. If your feet are uncomfortable and do not lay flat against the floor, place small rolled-up towels underneath them. See Figure 63. As you continue this exercise over time, make the rolls smaller until they are no longer needed.

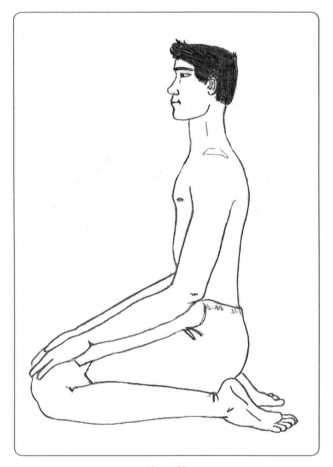

Figure 60

2 For recommended equipment, please see body4golf.com

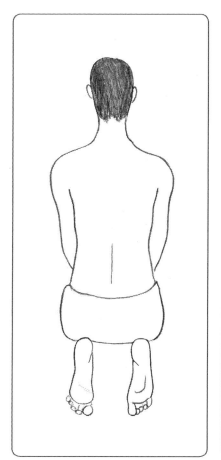

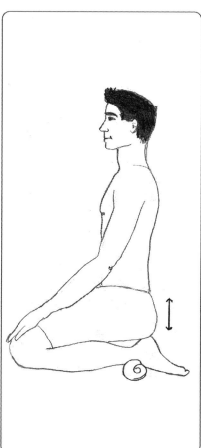

Left, Figure 61   Middle, Figure 62   Right, Figure 63

The HPLB complex appears to be the least understood and most overlooked area for improving golf performance. These three areas work together so intricately that it would be impossible to separate them for discussion, testing, improving ROM, or when trying to improve your golf swing.

For optimum performance with your golf swing, the pelvis needs to shift over the hips from right to left, and rotate right and then left over each hip/leg. See Figures 64, 65, 66, and 67. This is done in the closed-chain position—when the feet are touching the ground. During the swing, some golfers rotate their pelvis more than they shift it, and some golfers shift their pelvis more than they rotate it.

To learn more about the body mechanics of golf for this particular area, read this chapter's Testing/Concepts and Injury sections or, if you prefer, just skip to the exercises designed to regain any lost motion in this area.

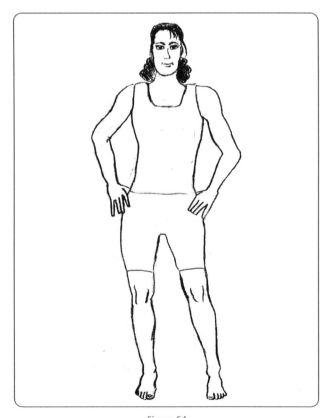

Figure 64

Testing/Concepts

The pelvis rotation and hip up/down tests are looking for the motion needed in your pelvis to shift and rotate. These motions occur through all phases of the golf swing beginning when moving from the stance phase to the backswing and ending with the follow-through.

For shifting and rotation of the pelvis over the hips to occur, the lumbar musculature and hip flexor muscle on one side of the body need to contract by shortening (concentrically) and on the other side need to contract by controlled lengthening (eccentrically). There are many muscles involved in pelvis motion during the golf swing. I am going to start by focusing on the hip flexors.

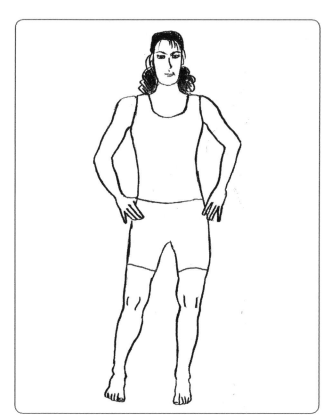

Figure 65

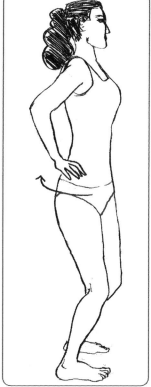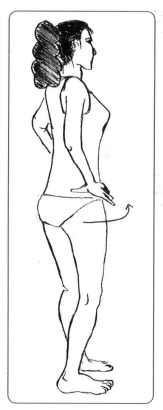

Left, Figure 66   Right, Figure 67

Note in Figure 68 the origins and insertion (the areas of bone the muscles attach to) of the two bellies of the hip flexor. The hip flexor muscle bellies start from the last thoracic vertebrae, the lumbar vertebrae and the large bony area of the pelvis and attach to the femur or thigh bone. This muscle crosses over every joint in the lumbar/pelvis/hip complex, making this muscle intricately involved in the motions needed for a good swing pattern.

This concept explains the selection of testing and exercises to improve maximum lumbar/pelvis/hip motion. The up-and-down motion of the pelvis over the hips, used for testing and

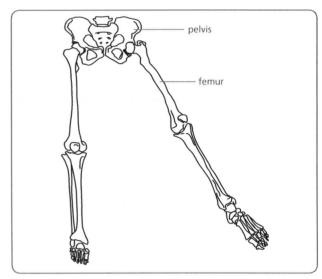

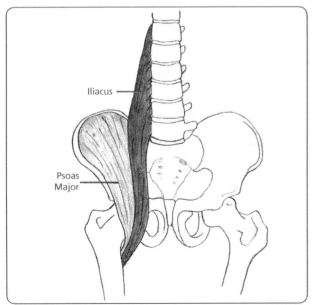

Figure 68

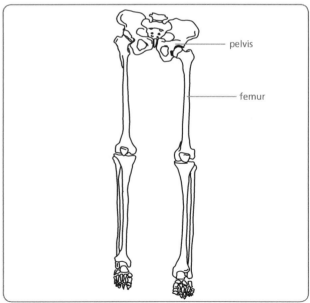

Top, Figure 69   Bottom, Figure 70

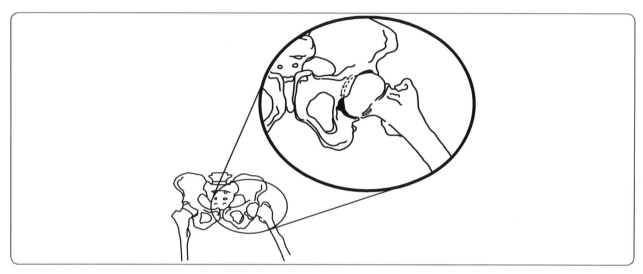

Figure 71

as a flexibility-improving movement exercise, appears to be a seemingly small motion, but requires the head of the femur (the ball of the long leg bone) to cover a large area of joint surface in the pelvis. Where the ball part of the leg bone and the socket part of the pelvis meet is commonly known as the hip joint. Abducting your hip (moving your leg out to the side) is shown in Figure 69. A large distance is traveled by the foot and a corresponding smaller distance moved at the hip joint. To drop one side of your pelvis and raise the other side over your hips, a smaller amount of body movement occurs with the same corresponding small distance moved at the hip joint. See Figure 70. The distances traveled by the head of the femur (the ball portion) in the pelvis (where the

socket is) for the femur moving in the pelvis, or the pelvis moving over the femur as pictured above in Figure 71 are comparatively equal. When you move the pelvis over the hip, you engage the entire lumbar/hip/pelvis complex and more accurately train for the goal of golf. This motion will relax and lengthen your hip flexors and lumbar musculature.

Every professional golfer that I have treated who is known for their beautiful swing had greater than what is considered normal pelvis/hip motion.

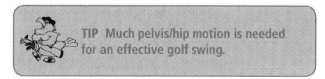

TIP Much pelvis/hip motion is needed for an effective golf swing.

The following figure represents an example of hip internal rotation. Try this yourself. Lie on the floor and roll the leg from the hip, in toward the midline. The shaded area on the diagram represents the area of the contracting muscles. See Figure 72. These are the inner thigh muscles and the front part of the gluteus (buttocks) musculature.

These are the same muscles that pull the pelvis around the fixed left leg in the follow-through phase of the swing. When the internal rotators contract, they cannot rotate the leg inward because the foot is fixed on the ground, so they pull the pelvis around the hip. See Figure 73. Figures 74 and 75 show the pelvis rotating over the leg.

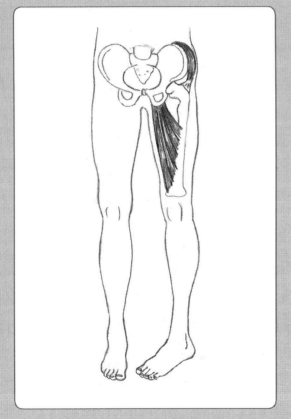

Figure 72

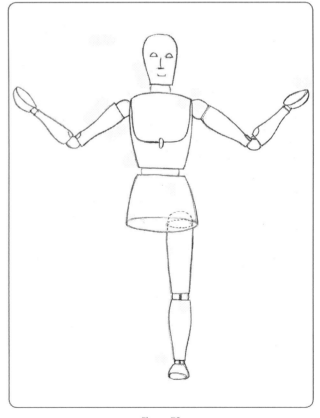

Figure 73

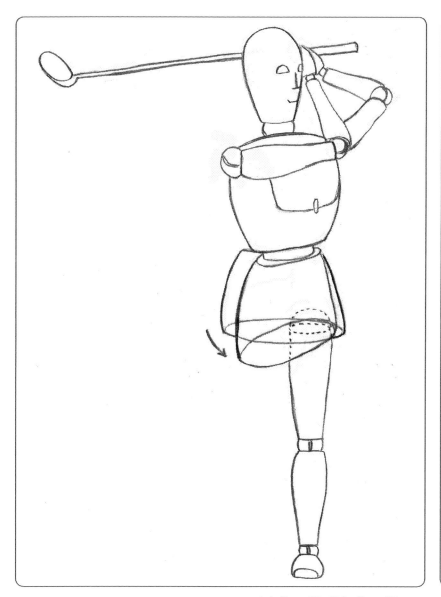

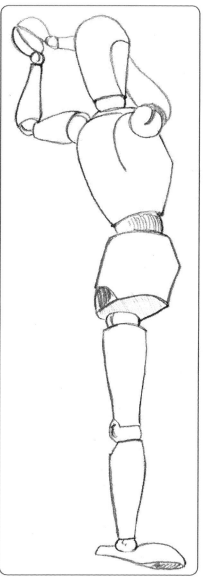

Left, Figure 74   Right, Figure 75

The Golfer's Prep

To better understand the golfer's prep, try standing up and moving your body as it is described below. Golfers prep their pelvis by rotating their pelvis to the right over the right leg during the backswing, prior to turning their pelvis left for the downswing, impact, and follow-through. See Figures 76 and 77. The twist to the right creates stored force that naturally wants to uncoil in the opposite direction. Think of a towel twisted taut. See Figures 78 and 79. When you let go of the towel, it automatically unravels in the opposite direction. This is what a golfer's pelvis does from backswing to follow-through. After storing the force by the pelvis rotating to the right for the backswing, the pelvis will unravel to the left. Golf instructors describe this pelvis and trunk rotation as being "wound," "coiled," or "stacked." It is not the stretch at the end that presets the muscles, but the lengthening and shortening contractions of pelvis and trunk musculature getting you into the position that gives you the stored force. If you are rotating your trunk and pelvis to the right until everything is stretched tight, you may be setting yourself up for injuries. For further information, read the gray box on page 64.

Not only is the pelvis important for motion, it is also the FOUNDATION and STABILITY for the trunk and upper extremities. Just as the foundation of a house supports the frame and walls, the hip/pelvis/low back complex supports the trunk and extremities. Unlike the foundation for a house, the hip/pelvis/low back complex is a dynamic or continuously moving foundation. It is important for this area to be stable and balanced while moving. Loss of ROM of the hip/pelvis/low back complex will influence the dynamic balance and stability of the golf swing and lead to many types of compensations. The two main compensations resulting from loss of ROM are dropping your buttocks closer to the ground to lower your center of gravity and shifting your pelvis more while exaggerating trunk side-bending. Both of these compensations increase your base of support, creating more stability.

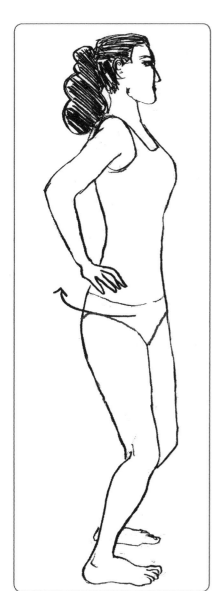
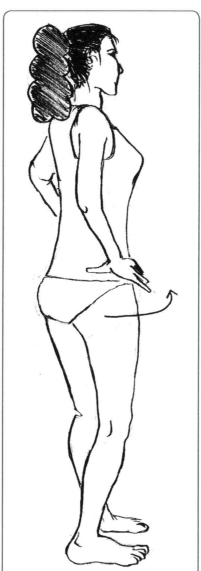
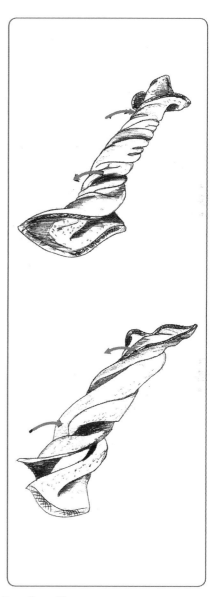

Left, Figure 76   Middle, Figure 77   Right Top, Figure 78   Right Bottom, Figure 79

During the swing, the pelvis rotates right over the right leg in a closed-chain position (feet on the floor), by contracting the right hip internal rotators. The left hip is now positioned with its hip internal rotators on stretch. The golfer then fires the left hip internal rotators and powerfully rotates the pelvis over the left leg. Hip rotator muscle pictures can be seen in Appendix B.

To take the golf prep a little further (and it does get complex), let's talk about what the hip external rotators are doing. When the golfer rotates his pelvis right over his left leg, his left leg external rotators are moving the pelvis over the left leg. Then the golfer fires the right hip external rotators to powerfully rotate the pelvis over the right leg.

The last step (and I may lose you here), would be to look at the two combined. As the golfer rotates his pelvis right, the following occurs: The right hip internal rotators contract concentrically, while the left hip internal rotators lengthen with eccentric control.

The left hip external rotators contract concentrically, while the right hip external rotators lengthen with eccentric control.

As the golfer powerfully rotates his pelvis left, the following occurs: The left hip internal rotators contract concentrically, while the right hip internal rotators lengthen with eccentric control.

The right hip external rotators contract concentrically, while the left hip external rotators lengthen with eccentric control.

If done properly, a golfer does a small prep of the pelvis over the legs to the right and then powerfully contracts and rotates the pelvis to the left. For the duration of the pelvic rotation motion, the right and left sides of the pelvis are working synchronously together.

Hip Internal Rotators
Adductor Longus
Adductor Brevis
Adductor Magnus
Anterior Gluteus Medius
Anterior Gluteus Minimus
Tensor Fasciae latae
Pectineus
Gracilis

Hip External Rotators
Gluteus Maximus
Obturator Internus
Obturator Externus
Quadratus Femoris
Piriformis
Gemellus Superior
Gemellus Inferior
Sartorius
Posterior Gluteus Medius

TIP The swing may start from the trunk, but the rotation of the body begins from the pelvis/hip musculature, specifically the left hip internal rotators and the right hip external rotators. This motion, if done properly, adds considerable power to the golf swing.

Injuries

This section combines normal results from biomechanical breakdown (joint motion) as well as observations I have made over the years in my clinic.

Because this area has such complex motion, initial loss of motion of one side generally results in pain on the opposite side, or restrictions in the front of the body (anterior) result in back of the body (posterior) pain and vice versa. There are numerous examples. For instance, loss of ROM of the right sacroiliac joint would present with left sacroiliac pain, loss of motion of the pubic symphysis would present with iliosacral pain, and a tightened iliacus portion of the hip flexor would result in iliosacral problems and pain. Once the pelvic area is severely compromised in motion, frequent problems are tight IT bands, patella tracking problems, groin pain, restrictions in the rib cage for breathing, and neck pain.

 TIP If your body is not capable of rotating left, you will need to shift your pelvis or weight to the left more and side-bend your trunk to the right to continue your swing.

 TIP Loss of ROM in the hip/pelvis/low back complex will influence the strength of your core (the trunk musculature). Every point where your pelvis is not moving smoothly and on a level plane as you swing is a point where your core is compromised, weak, or not functioning.

Exercises

The advanced hip up/down exercise and the pelvic figure eights exercise are both important and effective for coordinating and training the hips/pelvis/low back complex. These movement exercises help the right and left sides of the pelvis work together. Training this group of muscles as a unit will improve your golf swing. As motion is improved in these areas, there will be less compression at the sacroiliac (SI) joint, a common area for golfers to have problems.

Pictures of the hip internal rotator musculature and hip external rotator musculature are located in Appendix B.

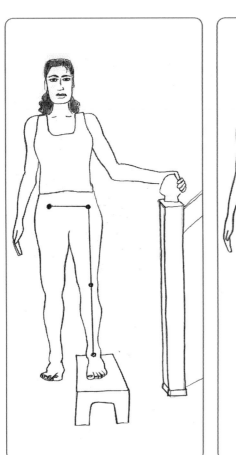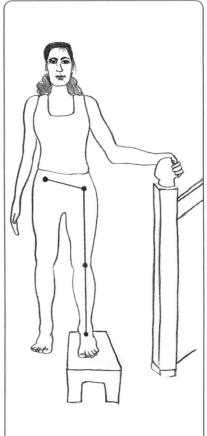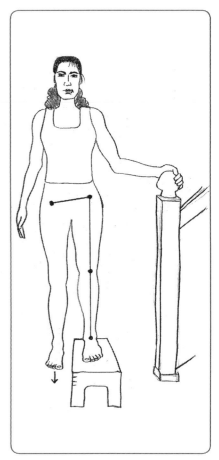

Left, Figure 80   Center, Figure 81   Right, Figure 82

Hip Ups/Hip Downs

Start this exercise by standing and placing your right foot on a stair or stool. Make sure your leg is straight under your pelvis. To do this, you must hold on to something. Now raise and lower your left pelvis. Your left leg should raise and lower with your pelvis. Make sure your pelvis is dropping straight and not rotating forward or backward. See Figures 80, 81, and 82. Repeat 4–12 times on each leg. This exercise will improve your hip flexor flexibility.

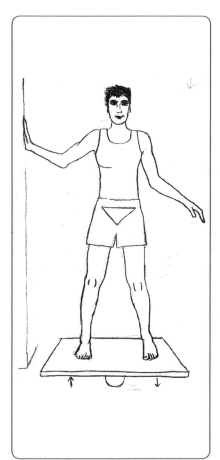 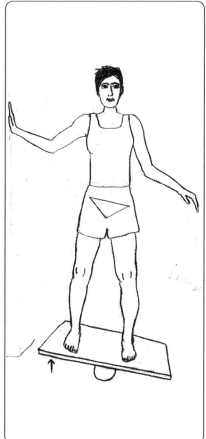 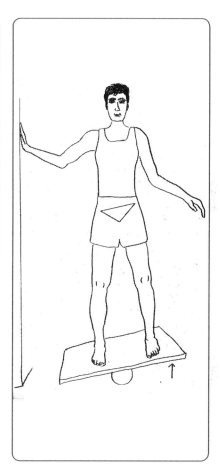

Left, Figure 83   Middle, Figure 84   Right, Figure 85

Advanced Hip Ups/Hip Downs

For this exercise, you will need a balance board. See body4golf.com for recommendations. Perform hip ups and downs on the board with your knees slightly bent. The knees stay fixed and will not bend or straighten. Make sure you have something to hold onto for balance. Optimally, you this exercise without holding on to anything for balance. See Figures 83, 84, and 85. Repeat 4–12 times.

Pelvic Figure Eights

Stand in a room with your back to a wall, and with walls to your right and left to be used as reference points. Place your feet 3–6 inches more than hip-distance apart. A good position to start would be your stance position. Your knees are bent and your back and neck are straight. Your hands will be at your waist with palms facing the floor. Your hands are in this position as a reminder to keep your pelvis level. Your feet will remain flat on the floor throughout the exercise and your knees will bend various amounts to keep your pelvis level. See Figure 86.

You will be mapping a figure eight with your pelvis. Start by facing forward. Begin moving your pelvis right along the pattern of the eight. As you start to shift your weight over your right leg, maximally rotate your pelvis until it faces the wall to your right. Do this by rotating your pelvis in a circle over your right leg. Next, begin moving your pelvis backward to the left. As your pelvis approaches the center of the figure eight, rotate back to neutral. You will again be facing forward or close to it. Then begin moving your pelvis left along the pattern of the eight. As you start to shift your weight over your left leg, maximally rotate your pelvis until it faces the wall to your left. Do this by rotating your pelvis in a circle over your left leg. Return back to the center of the eight. Continue the figure eights by flowing from right to left for 4–12 repetitions. Begin with larger eights for the first set, progressing to smaller eights for the last. This exercise can also be done in reverse. See Figures 87, 88, 89, 90, 91, 92, and 93.

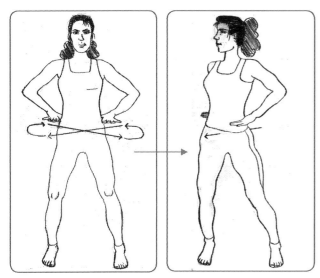

Left, Figure 86   Right, Figure 87

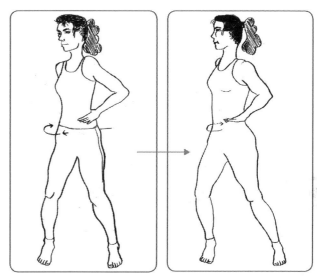

Left, Figure 88   Right, Figure 89

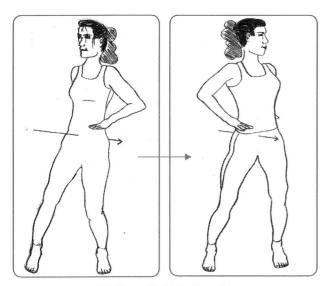

Left, Figure 90   Right, Figure 91

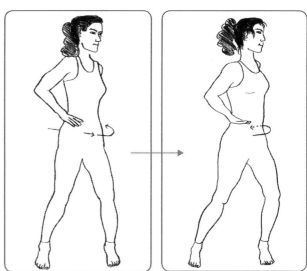

Left, Figure 92   Right, Figure 93

Standing Pelvic Tilts

The following movement is demonstrated for practice. It is used in many of the hip exercises to improve ROM. Stand with your feet hip-distance apart. Now tighten your lower abdomen and buttocks musculature, moving the bottom portion of your pelvis forward. This action flattens your lower back. This is a posterior pelvic tilt. See Figure 94.

Now reverse this by relaxing and lengthening the abdominal musculature and tightening the lower back musculature. This action arches your back and accentuates your buttocks. This is an anterior tilt. See Figure 95. Now move slowly back and forth between anterior and posterior tilting until you feel comfortable with this motion.

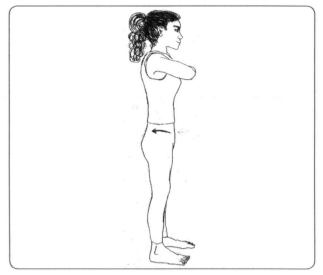

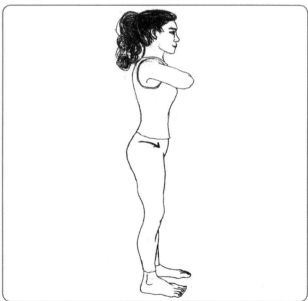

Top, Figure 94   Bottom, Figure 95

Hip Adductor Lengthening

Spread your legs apart, keeping your right foot pointing forward (perpendicular to your leg), and your left foot in the direction of the leg. Make sure your hip and knee on the left leg are aligned directly over the second toe. See Figure 96. Now bend the knee of the left leg, allowing your pelvis to drop down and toward the bent leg. Keep your legs and body in the same plane as in Figure 97. If you are having trouble keeping your body in one plane, start with your legs closer together. Move down until you feel resistance and then come back to the starting position. Resistance should be felt in the inner thigh area anywhere from the pelvis to the knee. Repeat 4–12 times each leg.

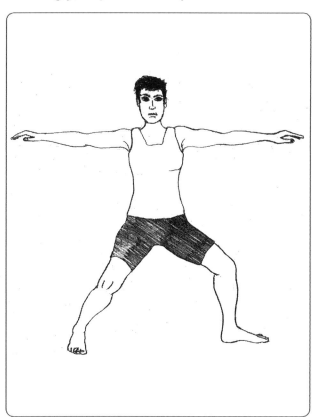

Figure 96

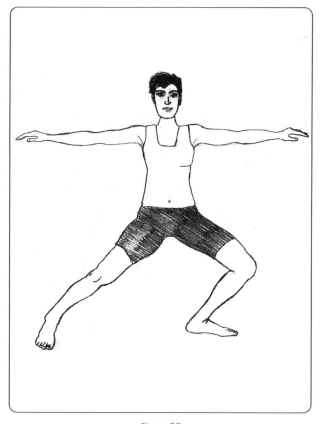

Figure 97

Pigeon Position

This stretch targets the outside of the thigh or iliotibial band, the pelvis musculature, and the pelvic floor musculature (a bowl-shaped group of muscles attaching to the bottom inside area of the pelvis). Begin by sitting with legs crossed. Move one leg out of the sit position, bringing it in backward underneath you. Make sure your pelvis and back are flat and level, feet are straight out from the legs, and arms are in front or to the side of you. See Figure 98. Relax over the bent leg by moving your pelvis backward with the leg. When you feel resistance, back off a little and begin to lengthen your legs away from the body in the direction they are placed. Lengthen your legs in the directions of the arrows on figure 99. This helps open the pelvis. You should feel resistance in the lower area of the pelvis or the outside of the bent leg. Now take a deep breath and let it out. Repeat taking breaths 4–12 times. This should feel the same on both sides. If one side is painful, do not do this exercise and consider seeking body work.

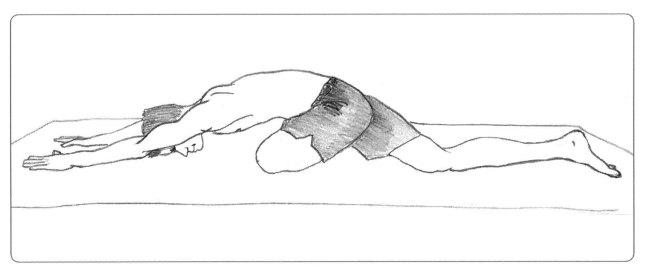

Figure 98

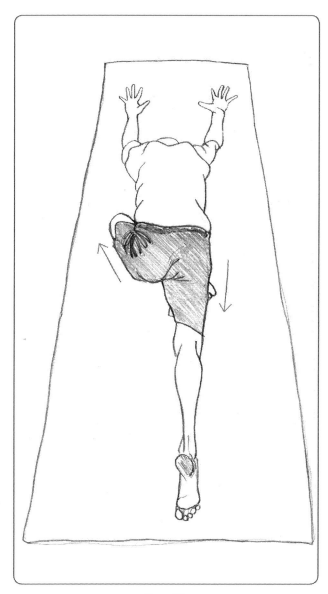

Figure 99

Quadriceps Lengthening

Stand straight with your right leg bent at the knee and your foot approaching your buttocks. See Figures 100 and 101. At the height of where your right foot falls, place it on a surface at this height. A couch, bed, or table works well. The foot should be pointed and in alignment with the leg. Make sure your legs are hip-distance apart and the knee is pointing straight down toward the floor. Your trunk is straight and your pelvis is level in a posterior tilt. If any of the alignment is hard, move farther away from the table or other surface to start. You may need something to hold on to. Now bring your whole trunk, pelvis, and hip back, moving the upper thigh as close to the lower leg as you can while still keeping alignment. Move until there is resistance, and then move forward again. Make sure that your knee continues to point straight down toward the floor and that you are not arching your back. If you can touch your foot to your buttocks while maintaining alignment, then bend the leg you are standing on at the knee by slightly squatting until you feel resistance and then straighten your leg. See Figure 102. The movement should be a small motion about 1–2 inches. Resistance should be felt in the front of the thigh anywhere from the pelvis to the knee, as well as possibly in the ankle. Repeat 4–12 times for each leg.

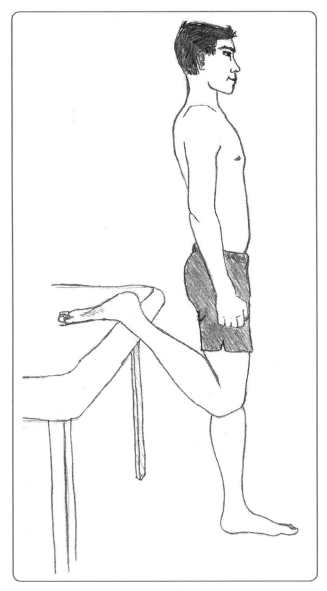

Figure 100

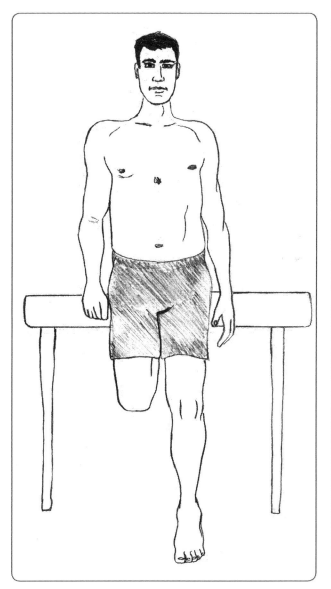

Figure 101

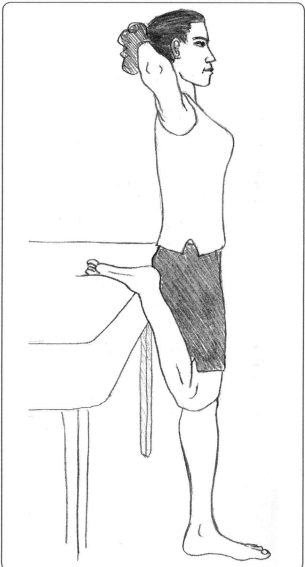

Figure 102

Hamstring Lengthening (Open Chain)

Stand placing your right leg up on a surface in front of you with your right foot pulled in toward you. Then position the left leg with the foot at a right angle. See Figure 103. Keep your pelvis neutral, not tilted from side to side or front to back. If you are not able to keep your pelvis neutral, then start with a lower surface, such as a chair, stool, or step. Rotate your trunk so that you are directly facing your outstretched leg. Hold your arms up straight from your body and arch toward your foot until you feel resistance, then move back to the starting position. See Figure 104. You should feel resistance in the back of the thigh anywhere from the pelvis to the knee. Repeat 4–12 times each leg.

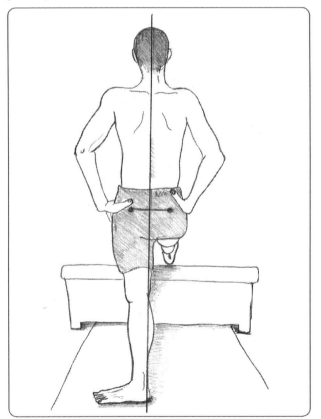

Figure 103

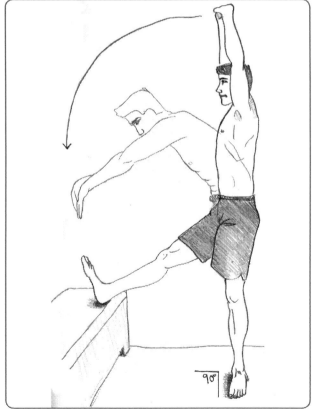

Figure 104

Chapter 4: **Exercises for the Hips/Pelvis/Low Back**

Hip Internal Rotators Lengthening (Open Chain)

Stand placing your right leg up on a surface in front of you with your right foot rotated out to the right side. To do this, rotate the right leg laterally from the hip or externally. Then position the left leg with the foot at a right angle. See Figure 105. Keep your pelvis neutral, not tilted from side to side or front to back. If you are not able to keep your pelvis neutral, then start with a lower surface, such as a chair, stool, or step. Rotate your trunk so that you are directly facing your outstretched leg. Hold your arms up straight from your body and arch toward your foot until you feel resistance, then move back to the starting position. See Figure 106. You may feel slight resistance. If there is no resistance, find a higher surface to place your foot on. If the starting position is difficult to achieve, choose a lower surface such as a step or small stool. Resistance should be felt in the lower pelvis, buttocks, or inner thigh area. Repeat 4–12 times each leg.

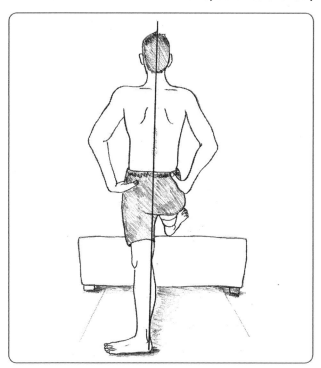

Figure 105

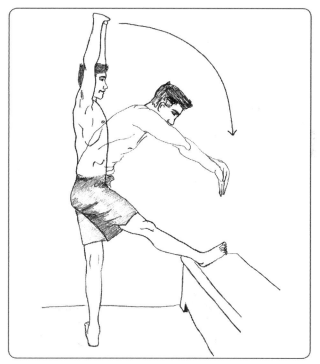

Figure 106

Hamstring Lengthening (Closed Chain)

Stand in front of a table or desk with your feet pointing forward. Spread your legs with right leg forward and left leg behind you with about a foot's distance between them. The right leg should be farther forward from your trunk than your left leg is backward. See Figures 107 and 108.

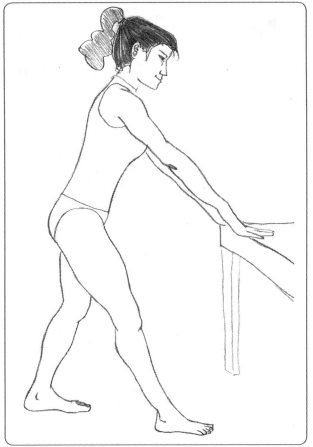

Figure 107

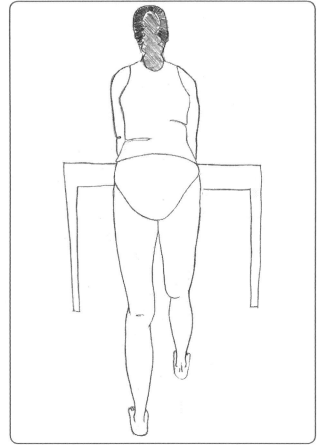

Figure 108

Now bend forward at the waist and place your hands on the surface you have chosen. A table works well. Keep your back flat and pelvis level. Now start those anterior and posterior tilts. See Figures 109 and 110. You should feel resistance in the right leg anywhere from the pelvis or buttocks area to the ankle. If there is no resistance, place your left leg farther back and repeat. If you are unable to do the pelvic tilts, bring your legs closer together by making the distance less than a foot and try again. Repeat 4–12 times each leg.

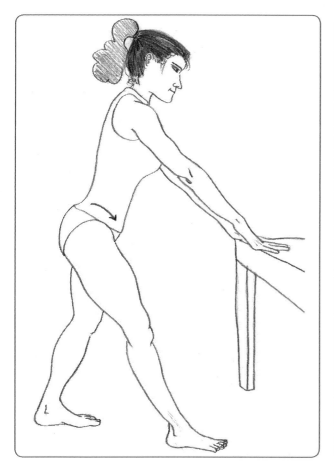

Figure 109

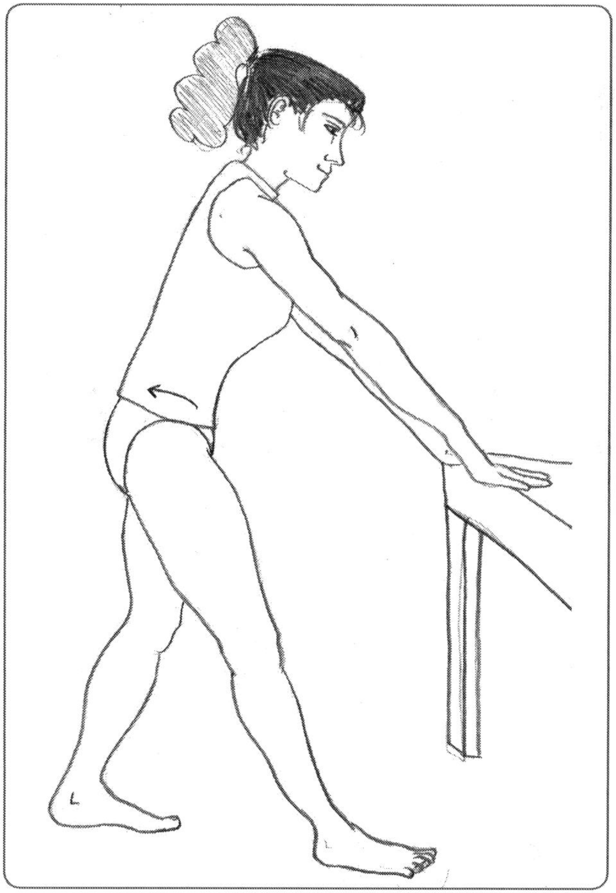

Figure 110

Hip Internal Rotator Lengthening (Closed Chain)

Stand in front of a table or desk with feet pointed forward. Spread your legs with your right leg forward and your left leg behind you with about a foot's distance between them. Your right leg should be farther forward from your trunk than your left leg is backward. Rotate the right leg out to the right or externally from the hip. See Figures 111 and 112.

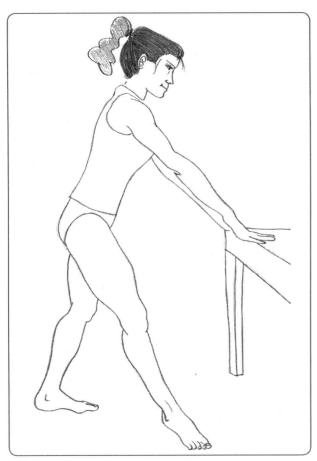

Figure 111

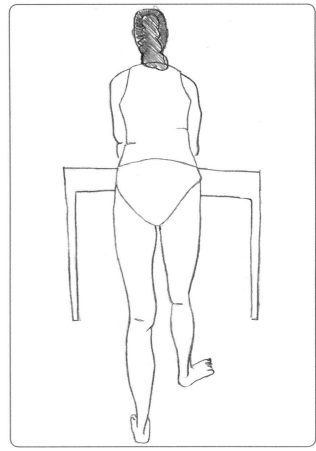

Figure 112

Now bend forward at the waist and place your hands on the surface you have chosen. Keep your back flat and pelvis level. Now start those anterior and posterior tilts. See Figures 113 and 114. You should feel resistance in the right leg buttocks area to the ankle. If there is no resistance, place your left leg farther back and repeat. If you are unable to do the pelvic tilts, bring your legs closer together by making the distance less than a foot and try again. Resistance should be felt in the lower pelvis, buttocks, or inner thigh area. Repeat 4–12 times each leg.

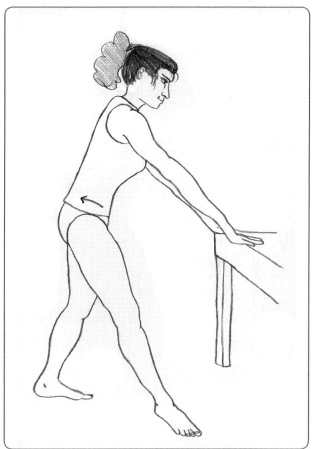

Figure 113

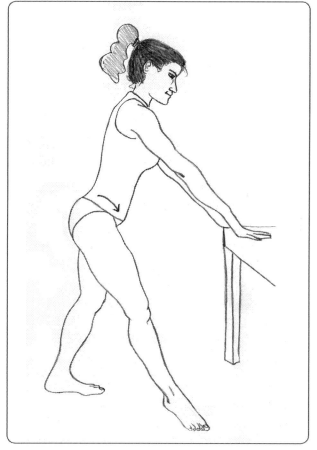

Figure 114

The amount of trunk rotation needed for the backswing and follow-through is immense. Therefore, keeping this area of your body moving well will help you go fluidly from backswing to follow-through. For the purpose of this book, the "trunk" will be defined as the shaded area in Figure 115. Trunk musculature will include the abdominal musculature, the spine musculature, and the rib cage musculature.

To learn more about the body mechanics of golf for this particular area, read this chapter's Testing/Concepts and Injury sections or, if you prefer, just skip to the exercises designed to regain any lost motion for this area.

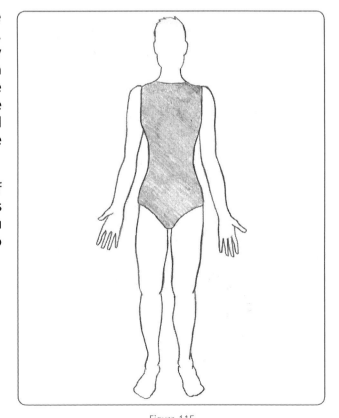

Figure 115

Testing/Concepts

Optimally, the rib cage should be long and tapered toward the waist with spaces in between each rib. See Figure 116. Often, however, rib cages are flared out above the waist with little rib spacing, and the chest is widened laterally or out to the sides. See Figure 117. The result of a more barrel-shaped chest, as pictured in Figure 117, is poor trunk rotational ROM, a weakened core from the abdominal musculature being lengthened, and poor shoulder and neck motion.

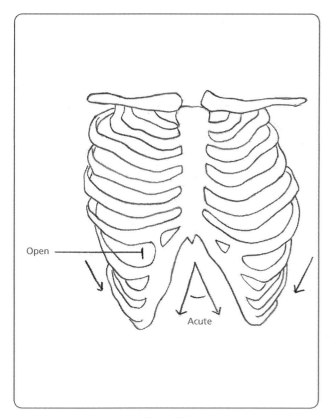

Figure 116

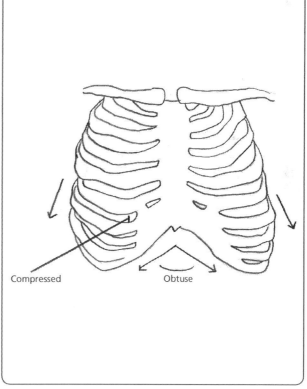

Figure 117

Because the golfer is holding a club with both hands, allowing the arms to move synchronously together, the primary musculature used for the swing is the trunk. This means that the trunk is the GENERATOR of the golf swing. As proof of this statement, try this test at home. Hold both hands together as in Figure 118 and have someone resist your movement while you take your arms from above your right shoulder toward your left hip. This can also be done using exercise tubing, by attaching the tubing behind you and pulling the tubing with both hands as described above. Do several repetitions. You should feel this in the abdominal area and trunk area.

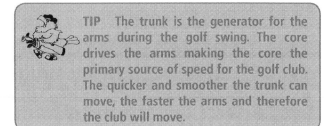

TIP   The trunk is the generator for the arms during the golf swing. The core drives the arms making the core the primary source of speed for the golf club. The quicker and smoother the trunk can move, the faster the arms and therefore the club will move.

As noted, the amount of trunk rotation needed for the backswing and follow-through is tremendous. The trunk begins rotating as your body leaves the stance phase, moves into the backswing, and then continues through the follow-through. The rib cage and thoracic vertebrae (the vertebrae that the ribs attach to) should provide a large portion of this motion. The more rotation provided by the rib cage

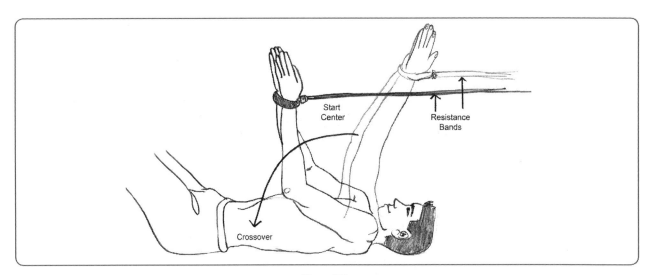

Start
Center

Resistance
Bands

Crossover

Figure 118

Chapter 5: Exercises for the Trunk/Rib cage

and thoracic vertebrae, the less the body will look for this motion in the lumbar vertebrae. This is good, as the five lumbar vertebrae are not structurally designed to rotate.

If the trunk does not rotate well, then the shoulder girdle (collarbone and shoulder blade) has to make up for this loss of ROM. To accommodate this extra motion needed from the shoulders, you will have to sacrifice quality of motion for quantity of motion. The positioning needed to supply extra motion places the clavicles and scapulas in positions with lengthened musculature, lengthened soft tissue, and therefore relatively poor strength. This concept is explained more thoroughly in Chapter 6: Exercises of the Upper Extremities (Arms). Often, golfers with poor rib cage motion will present with shoulder, wrist, and elbow problems.

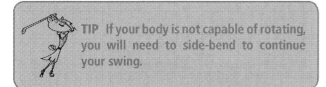

TIP If your body is not capable of rotating, you will need to side-bend to continue your swing.

When the trunk motion is restricted, the swing pattern can become fractured, causing you to lose your core. Picture this scenario: You rotate your trunk to the right for the backswing and when your trunk stops, you continue your arms farther up and back so the arms are positioned in what is considered a good backswing

position. Now you start your downswing with your arms moving and your trunk static. At this point, your core will be dysfunctional or nonfunctioning. As the arms catch up to the place where the trunk stopped moving, the trunk can begin its generator job. Basically, you have no core or trunk assistance for the beginning of the swing.

In this second scenario, you rotate your trunk to the right for the backswing and when your trunk stops you continue your arms farther up and back so the arms are positioned in what is considered a good backswing position. Then you start your trunk moving first. Since the arms began positioned farther back with excessive separation from the trunk, they will have to play catch-up. Since it is impossible for them to completely catch up to the trunk, they will end up behind you at club impact. In this scenario, you sacrifice shoulder strength and proper coordination with your trunk, so you look like you begin the downswing from the proper position. You also put yourself at risk for shoulder and wrist injuries.

TIP Arm and trunk motion need to coordinate. The trunk, or core, should be dynamic, or constantly moving, throughout the swing.

At the point in the downswing when the arms become fractured from the trunk, the body will try to compensate by contracting your lower abdominals. This will result in the entire trunk moving forward toward the ground, creating one of two possible scenarios. Either you will hit more fat shots bringing your club over the ball at an angle, or you will have to side-bend your trunk after the point where your arms catch up to your trunk to compensate for the earlier forward bending. Also, the side-bending may occur at a place in the swing where it was not intended.

 TIP Do not carry your golf bag, luggage, or briefcase over your shoulder. As you breathe out, the bag's weight presses down on the ribs. This weighted downward pressure causes the ribs to stick in the end range of breathing or expiration. In my practice, I have evaluated many golfers with their right shoulder lower than their left. After restoring the upper three ribs' proper motion for breathing, the shoulders miraculously sit at the same height. (And you thought the unlevel shoulder was from the golf swing!)

 TIP The trunk and pelvis should initiate the golf swing. The core and HPLB complex team up to provide your power for the golf swing, fueling both the downswing (or acceleration of the club) and the backswing (or deceleration of the club).

Injuries

This section combines normal results from biomechanical breakdown (joint motion) as well as observations I have made over the years in my clinic.

Rib cage restrictions can cause various shoulder problems, neck pain, and headaches. Golfing with rib cage restrictions puts you at risk for rotator cuff tears. Another dysfunction created from golfing with a restricted rib cage is bilateral anterior positioned humeruses with facilitated biceps on the left arm and facilitated triceps on the right arm. Facilitated muscles present as constantly tight. You may develop shoulder calcific tendonitis or other bony changes to the acromioclavicular joint. If you swing with your trunk, you will injure yourself at the place your trunk stops moving or where core strength is challenged. At the point your trunk stops moving, one or both arms will bend at the elbow or your shoulders will change positions to continue the swing. At the point where your elbows bend uncontrollably, you will injure your shoulders.

 TIP The most critical place to lose trunk or core strength due to lack of trunk rotation or pelvis stability is at impact. At this critical place, you will injure primarily your left wrist.

Exercises

Trunk Rotation

Sit up straight in a chair with your legs crossed at the knees. See Figure 119. Rotate your trunk and head to the right. Remain upright as you rotate. Place your left arm on the right side of your legs. Push your left arm into your knees, to further your rotation. See Figure 120. Allow your right arm to rotate stretched out straight behind you. Rotate until you feel slight resistance in the trunk area. Take a deep breath, holding for a few seconds and then letting it out. Repeat breathing 4–12 repetitions. Then repeat, rotating left and taking 4–12 breaths. See Figures 121 and 122.

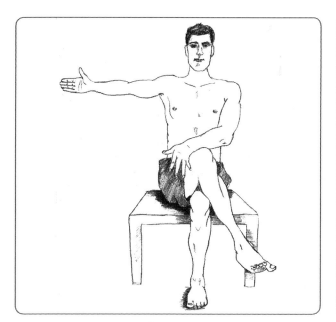

Figure 119

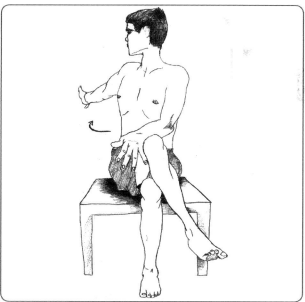

Figure 120

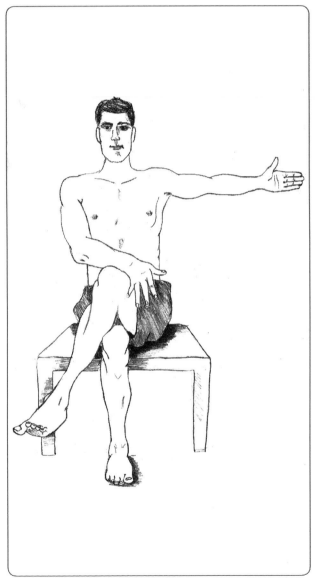

Figure 121

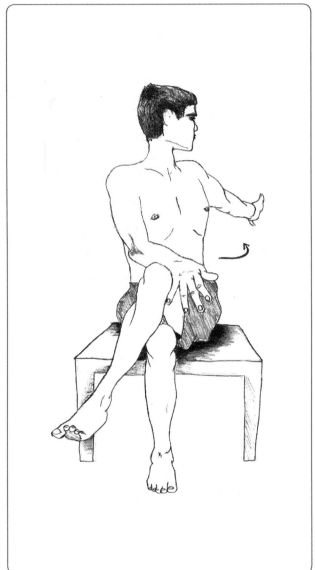

Figure 122

Chapter 5: Exercises for the Trunk/Rib cage

Trunk Side-Bending

Sit up straight with your feet flat. Drop your right shoulder down as low as it will go. Raise your left shoulder up as high as it will go. Let your head bend to the right side. See Figure 123. Take a deep breath, holding for a few seconds and then letting it out. Repeat breathing 10 times. Then drop your left shoulder down as low as it will go. Raise your right shoulder up as high as it will go. Let your head bend to the left side. See Figure 124. Take a deep breath, holding for a few seconds and then letting it out. Repeat breathing 4–12 times.

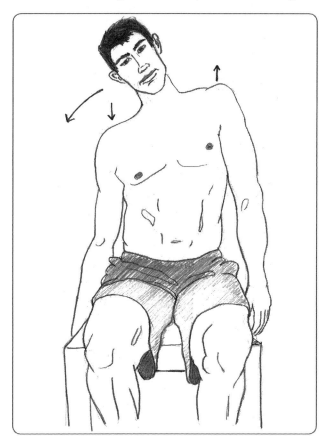

Figure 123

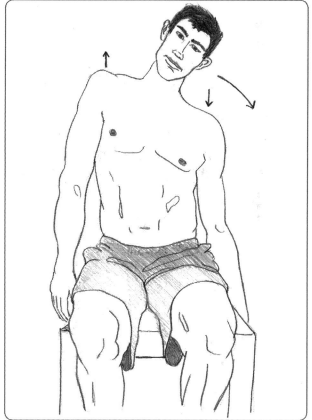

Figure 124

Upward/Downward Dog

Start on all fours with legs hip-distance apart and arms shoulder-distance apart. See Figure 125. Keep your back flat. Now rock back on your feet, moving them so that the bottoms are flat on the floor and bringing your body into an upside-down V. See Figure 126.

Your pelvis should lift up into the top of the V. Try to keep your legs straight and your back straight. Keep your back in line with your arms and your neck straight. Only move as far into the V as you can keep the legs and back straight and the feet flat. Then drop your abdomen toward the floor, letting your head move up toward the ceiling by rolling over your feet again. You will be allowing your belly to curve toward the floor and your back to arch up. Feet are in a ballet point. Chin is tucked. See Figure 127. Optimally, you should use your core to lift and lower the body while moving from downward to upward dog and back to downward dog. Continue up and down for 4–12 repetitions.

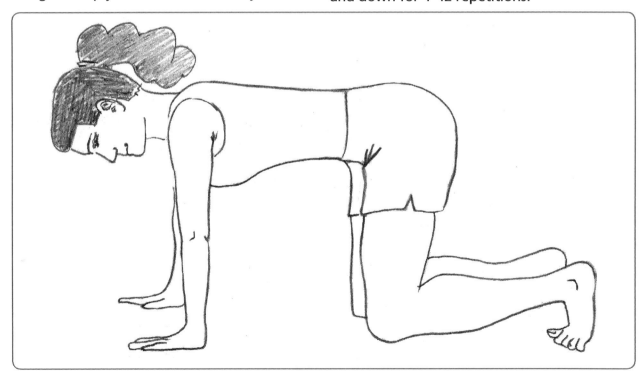

Figure 125

Chapter 5: Exercises for the Trunk/Rib cage

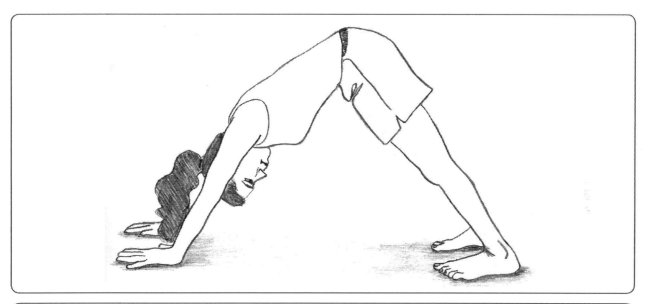

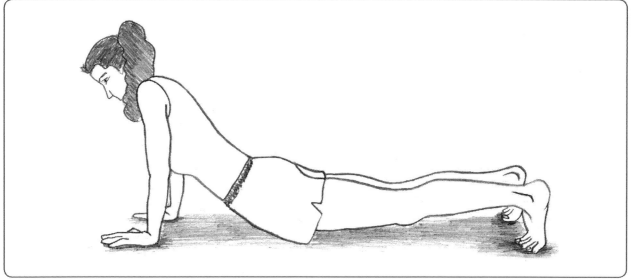

Top, Figure 126   Bottom, Figure 127

Sternum Raises

Your sternum is your breast bone in the front of your chest area. Sit with your hands behind your back. Pinch your scapulas in toward your spine and down toward the floor. See Figure 128. Now breathe into the upper part of your chest, lifting your sternum toward your nose. See Figure 129. Make sure you are keeping your head straight and your chin tucked. Repeat 4–12 times.

Upper Rib cage Lengthening

This exercise can be divided into three progressing modifications, or phases. The full exercise, Phase 3, is listed first, followed by Phases 1 and 2.

Phase 3: You will need a bench or large ottoman for this exercise. A corner of a bed may work. Lie down on your back with your head close enough to the end of the bench to move your arms off the bench. Bend your knees and keep your feet flat. Clasp your hands together at your abdomen with your elbows bent at a 90-degree angle. See Figure 130. Now flatten your rib cage and back toward the bench. You may keep your back slightly arched if that is more comfortable. Bring your lower ribs in toward your midline by tightening your abdominal muscles. Be careful not to lock the lower rib cage down so tightly that you cannot rotate properly through this area. See Figure 131.

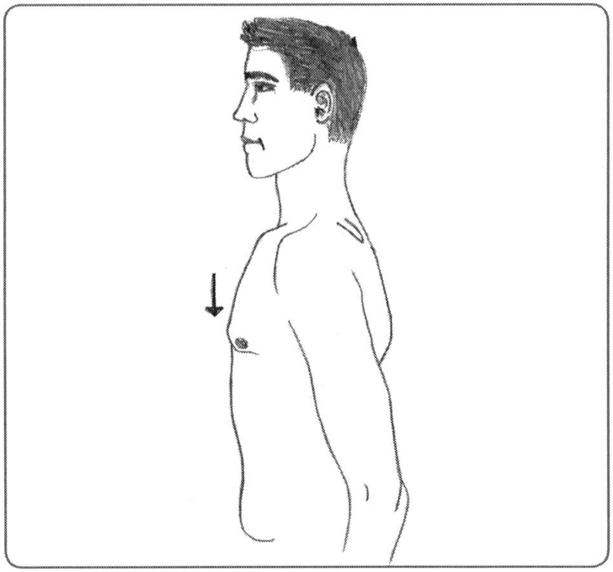

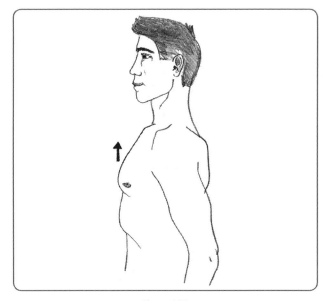

Figure 128

Figure 129

Hold your abdominals and lower ribs in this position, and lift your feet off the bench to engage your core. Then bring your hands over your head and down to the floor. Keep your elbows close together. As you move your arms, breathe into the upper ribs, moving your sternum toward your nose. As you let the breath out, lower your arms back to the bench. Continue to hold the lower rib and abdominal positions fixed as you do 4–12 repetitions of upper rib breathing with arm motion.

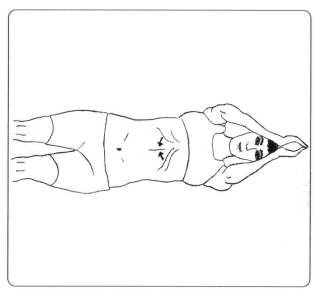

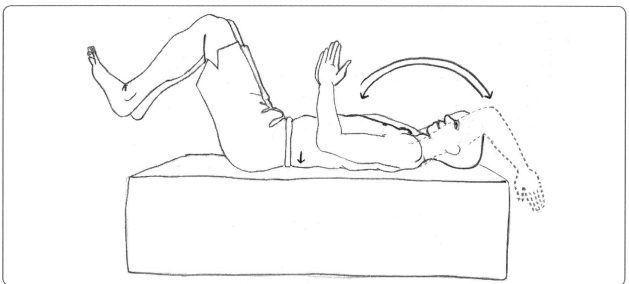

Top, Figure 131, Bottom Figure 130

Phase 1: You will need a bench or large ottoman for this exercise. A corner of a bed may work. Lie down on your back with your head close enough to the end of the bench to move your arms off the bench. Bend your knees and keep your feet flat. Clasp your hands together at your abdomen with your elbows bent at a 90-degree angle. Relax your upper arms by laying them on the bench. See Figure 132. Now flatten your rib cage and back toward the bench. You may keep your low back area slightly arched if that is more comfortable. Bring your lower ribs in toward your midline by tightening your abdominal muscles. See Figure 133. Be careful not to lock the lower rib cage down so tightly that you cannot rotate properly through this area. Hold your abdominals and lower ribs in this position and lift your feet off the bench to engage your core. Continue to lower and lift your feet off the bench holding your core. Do 4–12 repetitions.

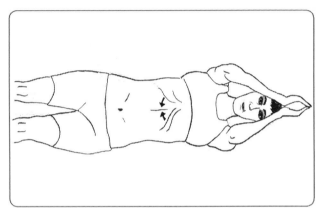

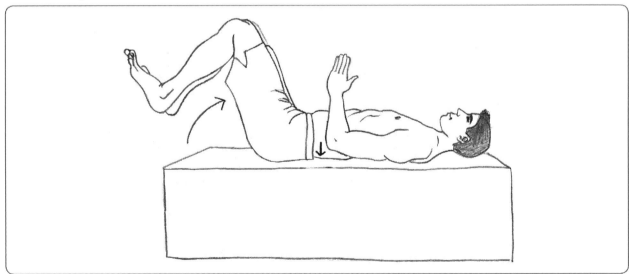

Top, Figure 133   Bottom, Figure 132

Chapter 5: **Exercises for the Trunk/Rib cage**

Phase 2, Part 1: You will need a bench or large ottoman for this exercise. A corner of a bed may work. Lie down on your back with your head close enough to the end of the bench to move your arms off the bench. Bend your knees and keep your feet flat. Clasp your hands together at your chest with your elbows bent at a 90-degree angle. See Figure 134. Now flatten your rib cage and back toward the bench. You may keep your back slightly arched if that is more comfortable. Bring your lower ribs in toward your midline by tightening your abdominal muscles. See Figure 135. Be careful not to lock the lower rib cage down so tightly that you cannot rotate properly through this area. Then bring your hands over your head and down to the floor. Keep your elbows close together and bent at a 90-degree angle. As you move your arms, breathe into the upper ribs, moving your sternum toward your nose. As you let the breath out, lower your arms back to the bench. Do 4–12 repetitions.

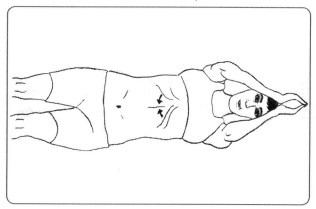

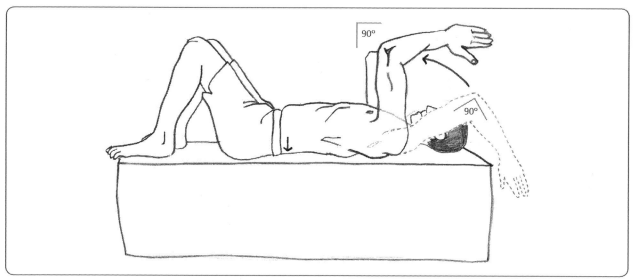

Top, Figure 135   Bottom, Figure 134

Phase 2, Part 2: You will need a bench or large ottoman for this exercise. A corner of a bed may work. Lie down on your back with your head close enough to the end of the bench to move your arms off the bench. Bend your knees and keep your feet flat. Clasp your hands together at your abdomen with your elbows bent at a 90-degree angle. Relax your upper arms by laying them on the bench. See Figure 136. Now flatten your rib cage and back toward the bench. Bring your lower ribs in toward your midline by tightening your abdominal muscles. See Figure 137. You may keep your back slightly arched if that is more comfortable. Be careful not to lock the lower rib cage down so tightly that you cannot rotate properly through this area. Hold your abdominals and lower ribs in this position and lift your feet off the bench to engage your core. Now breathe into the upper ribs, moving your sternum toward your nose. Continue to hold the lower legs up as you breathe in and out. Do 4–12 repetitions.

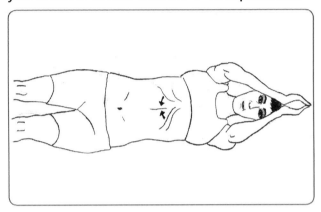

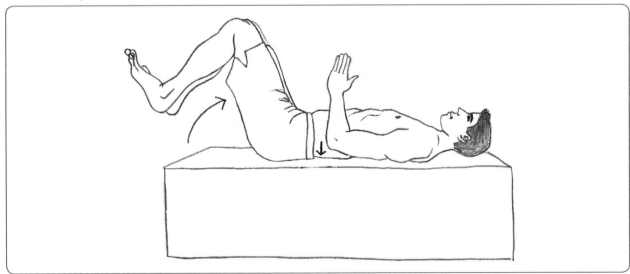

Top, Figure 137   Bottom, Figure 136

Chapter 5: **Exercises for the Trunk/Rib cage**

Modification of Upper Rib cage Lengthening (Done in Sitting)

If you still are having difficulty with this exercise, try performing it while sitting down. Sit in a comfortable chair with your arms at your side and your hands clasped together. Your elbows will be bent at a 90-degree angle. Flatten your back to the chair and pull your lower ribs together, engaging the abdominals and low back musculature. You may keep your back slightly arched if that is more comfortable. Be careful not to lock the

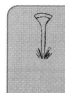

TIP   It is important to keep your upper rib-cage area (from the shoulders to about the fifth rib) flexible. Much shoulder musculature attaches to these ribs. Upper rib cage flexibility will allow more combined trunk rotation and shoulder flexibility for the backswing and follow-through phases of the golf swing.

lower rib cage down so tightly that you cannot rotate properly through this area. Raise your arms over your head, keeping your elbows at a 90-degree angle while breathing into your upper ribs and sternum. Do 4–12 repetitions. See Figures 138 and 139.

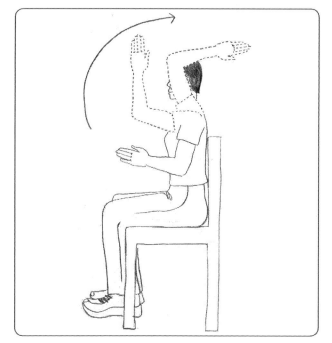

Figure 138

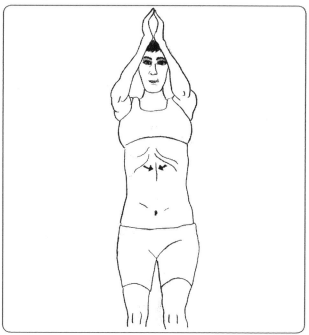

Figure 139

Chapter 6: Exercises for the Upper Extremeties (Arms)

The upper extremities guide and maneuver the club. The arms ensure the club face contacts the ball correctly. The arms can also increase the club speed by quickly straightening the elbows or moving the wrists, making the arms the secondary source of speed. Although the trunk is the primary musculature for the golf swing, arm strength is still necessary for an effective swing. The upper extremities are the most understood area of the body for golfing, and the most noticed area of the body for the golf swing. It is very easy to notice when your arms are not in the proper backswing position: Right arm around shoulder height rotated backward with the elbow bent and the left arm coming all the way across your body. It's also easy to notice your wrist not cocked properly or not moving to get to the impact position. The two tests for arms in this book were designed to determine the above ROM needs. The left arm coming across your body is indirectly tested with the "prayer behind the back" test.

To learn more about the body mechanics of golf for this particular area, read this chapter's Testing/Concepts and Injury sections or, if you prefer, just skip to the exercises designed to regain any lost motion in this area.

Testing/Concepts

Maximum strength of the shoulder and therefore the arms occurs with a stable scapula position. The scapula is most stable lying flat against the rib cage, retracted toward the spine, and slightly inferior or depressed. See Figure 140. This can be tested. Sit with your arm extended in front of you and lengthened as far forward as you can. Have someone try to push your arm down. See Figure 141. Now, keep your arm out but pull the scapula in toward your spine and down toward the floor. Have someone try to push your arm down again. See Figure 142. The second position with the scapula in its stable position should have resulted in a stronger arm.

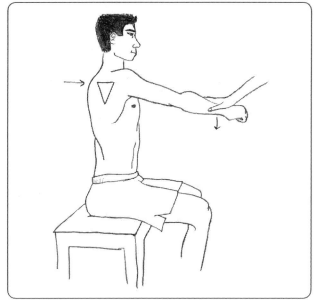

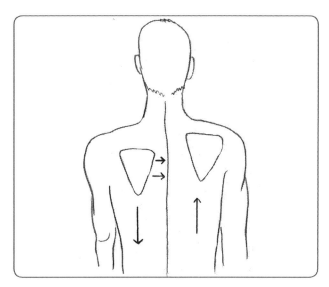

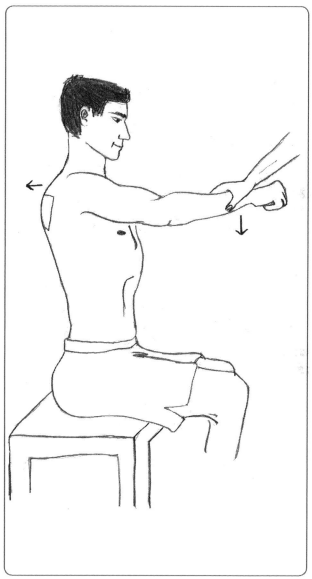

Top, Figure 140   Bottom, Figure 141

Figure 142

TIP If you are hitting a lot of fat shots, get your arm massaged. See the shaded area in Figure 143.

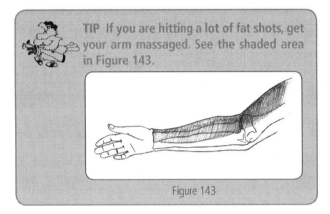

Figure 143

Injuries

This section combines normal results from biomechanical breakdown (joint motion) as well as observations I have made over the years in my clinic.

As mentioned earlier in the book, forearm injuries can result from fat shots. If the forearm area ROM is not regained, eventually you will have pain and dysfunction in the wrist, thumb, shoulder, and ribs. If you are a trunk swinger, you will present with upper rib problems or posterior positioned ribs from chronic loss of ROM in the shoulders and arms. If you are an arm swinger, you will present with facilitated pectoralis major, pectoralis minor, and subclavicular musculature. Facilitated muscles present as constantly tight.

Exercises

Upper Rib cage Lengthening

This exercise can be divided into three progressing modifications, or phases. The full exercise, Phase 3, is listed first, followed by Phases 1 and 2.

Phase 3: You will need a bench or large ottoman for this exercise. A corner of a bed may work. Lie down on your back with your head close enough to the end of the bench to move your arms off the bench. Bend your knees and keep your feet flat. Clasp your hands together at your chest with your elbows bent at a 90-degree angle. See Figure 144. Now flatten your rib cage and back toward the bench. You may keep your back slightly arched if that is more comfortable. Bring your lower ribs in toward your midline by tightening your abdominal muscles. See Figure 145. Be careful not to lock the lower rib cage down so tightly that you cannot rotate properly through this area. Hold your abdominals and lower ribs in this position, and lift your feet off the bench to engage your core.

Then bring your hands over your head and down to the floor. Keep your elbows close together. As you move your arms, breathe into the upper ribs, moving your sternum toward your nose. As you let the breath out, lower your arms back to the bench. Continue to hold the lower rib and abdominal positions fixed as you do 4–12 repetitions of upper rib breathing with arm motion.

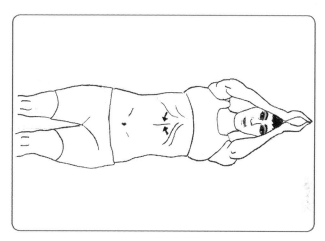

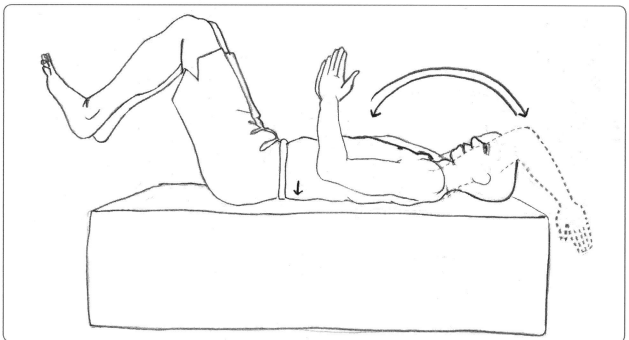

Bottom, Figure 144   Top, Figure 145

Phase 1: You will need a bench or large ottoman for this exercise. A corner of a bed may work. Lie down on your back with your head close enough to the end of the bench to move your arms off the bench. Bend your knees and keep your feet flat. Clasp your hands together at your abdomen with your elbows bent at a 90-degree angle. Relax your upper arms by laying them on the bench. See Figure 146. Now flatten your rib cage and back toward the bench. You may keep your low back area slightly arched if that is more comfortable. Bring your lower ribs in toward your midline by tightening your abdominal muscles. See Figure 147. Be careful not to lock the lower rib cage down so tightly that you cannot rotate properly through this area. Hold your abdominals and lower ribs in this position and lift your feet off the bench to engage your core. Continue to lower and lift your feet off the bench holding your core. Do 4–12 repetitions.

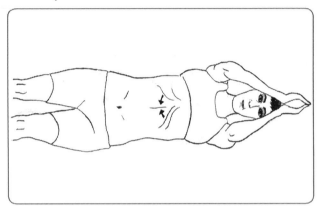

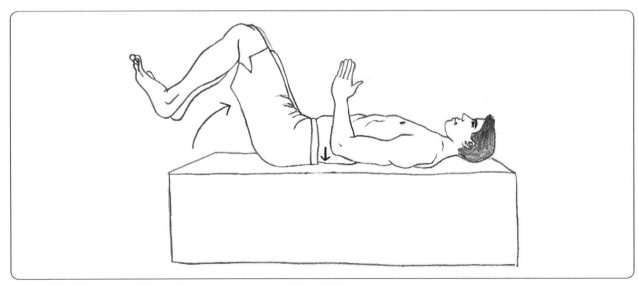

Top, Figure 147   Bottom, Figure 146

Chapter 6: **Exercises for the Upper Extremeties (Arms)**

Phase 2, Part 1: You will need a bench or large ottoman for this exercise. A corner of a bed may work. Lie down on your back with your head close enough to the end of the bench to move your arms off the bench. Bend your knees and keep your feet flat. Clasp your hands together at your chest with your elbows bent. See Figure 148. Now flatten your rib cage and back toward the bench. You may keep your back slightly arched if that is more comfortable. Bring your lower ribs in toward your midline by tightening your abdominal muscles. See Figure 149. Be careful not to lock the lower rib cage down so tightly that you cannot rotate properly through this area. Then bring your hands over your head and down to the floor. Keep your elbows close together and bent at a 90-degree angle. As you move your arms, breathe into the upper ribs, moving your sternum toward your nose. As you let the breath out, lower your arms back to the bench. Do 4–12 repetitions.

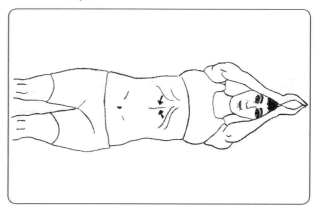

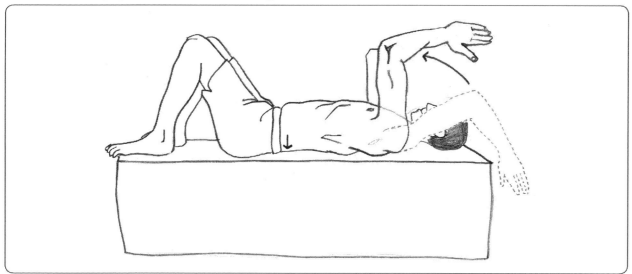

Top, Figure 149   Bottom, Figure 148

Phase 2, Part 2: You will need a bench or large ottoman for this exercise. A corner of a bed may work. Lie down on your back with your head close enough to the end of the bench to move your arms off the bench. Bend your knees and keep your feet flat. Clasp your hands together at your abdomen with your elbows bent at a 90-degree angle. Relax your upper arms by laying them on the bench. See Figure 150. Now flatten your rib cage and back toward the bench. Bring your lower ribs in toward your midline by tightening your abdominal muscles. See Figure 151. You may keep your back slightly arched if that is more comfortable. Be careful not to lock the lower rib cage down so tightly that you cannot rotate properly through this area. Hold your abdominals and lower ribs in this position and lift your feet off the bench to engage your core. Now breathe into the upper ribs, moving your sternum toward your nose. Continue to hold the lower legs up as you breathe in and out. Do 4–12 repetitions.

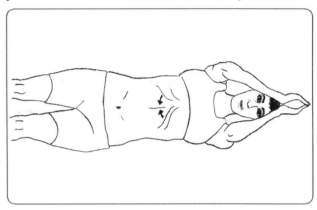

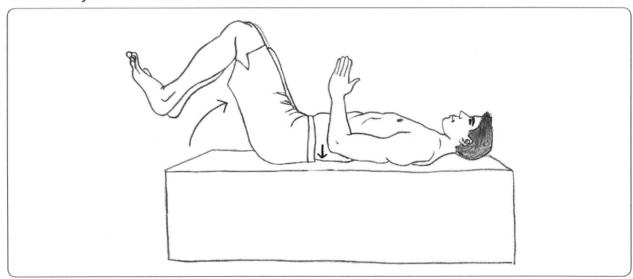

Top, Figure 151 Bottom, Figure 150

Chapter 6: **Exercises for the Upper Extremeties (Arms)**

Modification of Upper Rib cage Lengthening (Done in Sitting)

If you are still having difficulty with this exercise, try performing it while sitting down. Sit in a comfortable chair with your arms at your side and your hands clasped together. Your elbows will be bent at a 90-degree angle. Flatten your back to the chair and pull your lower ribs together, engaging the abdominals and low back musculature. You may keep your back slightly arched if that is more comfortable. Be careful not to lock the lower rib cage down so tightly that you cannot rotate properly through this area. Raise your arms over your head, keeping your elbows at a 90-degree angle while breathing into your upper ribs and sternum. Do 4–12 repetitions. See Figures 152 and 153.

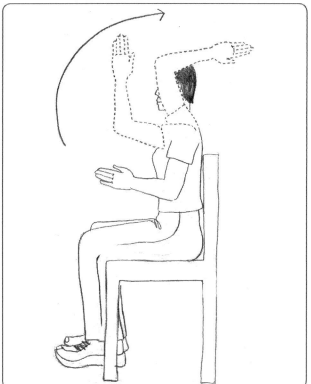

Figure 152

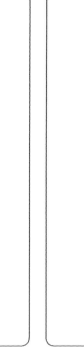

Figure 153

Quadruped Circles

Start by getting on your hands and knees, as in Figure 154. Keep your arms shoulder-distance apart and your legs hip-distance apart. Keep your palms flat on the floor. Shift your weight so that your arms are taking most of the load, and then start moving your entire body (as a unit) over your hands. This will move the arms in small circles over the hands. See Figures 155, 156. If you cannot keep your palms flat, then place small rolled up towels under your hands. Over time, decrease the size of the rolls until they are no longer needed. Repeat circles 4–12 repetitions.

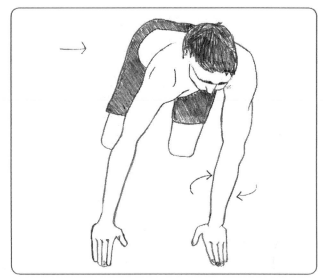

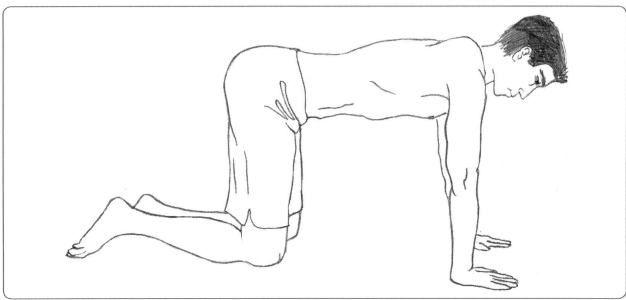

Top, Figure 155   Bottom, Figure 154

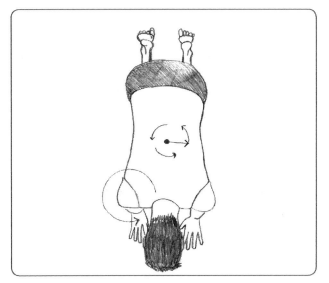

Figure 156

Body Bridging

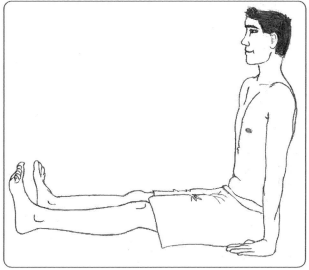

Start by sitting on the floor with your legs straight and your palms flat on the floor beside you, as in Figure 157. Roll up onto your feet, making a large bridge with your body. Keep your trunk, pelvis, upper legs, and neck straight. See Figure 158. Come back down to floor. Repeat 4–12 times.

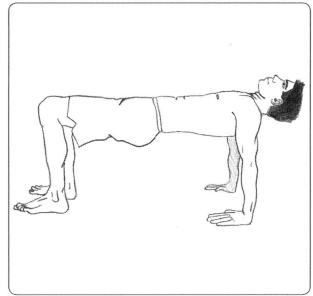

Top, Figure 157   Bottom, Figure 158

Prayer Position

If your result for the "prayer behind the back" test was poor, do not do this exercise. Start with the other exercises in this chapter and retest occasionally.

Start by sitting, placing your hands palm-to-palm behind your back in a reverse prayer position. See Figure 159. Now roll your hands in toward your spine until they are in a prayer position behind your back. See Figure 160. Your hands may separate to accomplish this. Move praying hands up your back. See Figure 161. Repeat 4–12 times.

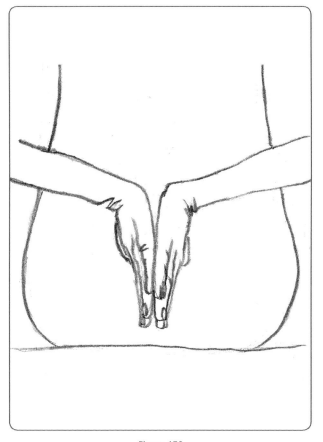

Figure 159

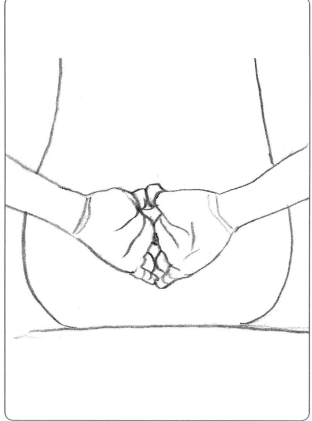

Figure 160

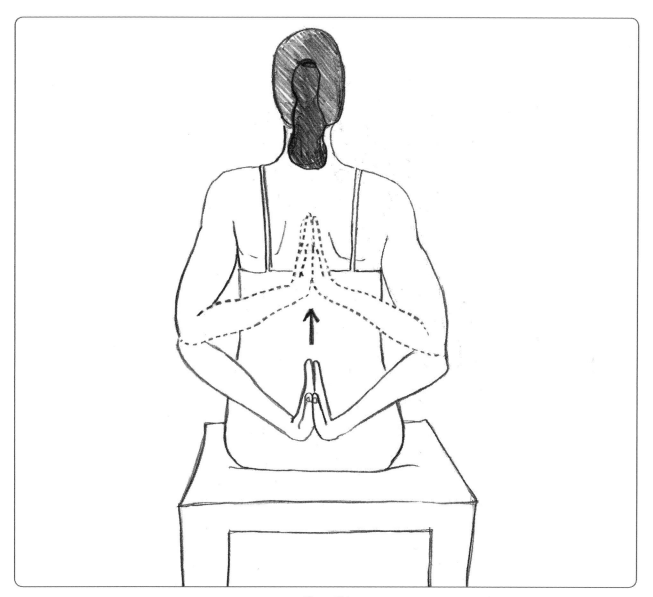

Figure 161

Chapter 7: Super Seven Warm-Up Exercises

Congratulations! If you're reading this chapter it means you have scored all GOOD and BEST on the ROM tests. To ensure you stay in peak form, consider doing the seven exercises listed below. These "Super Seven," as I like to call them, beautifully target the four areas of the body engaged in the golf swing and will ensure that you are warmed up and ready to play.

Three-Way Ankle

Setup is just like the test. Start by taking your knees forward, then equally to the right, then forward again, and then equally to the left. Repeat 4–12 times. There is no need to force motion at the end range, just keep moving. See Figure 162.

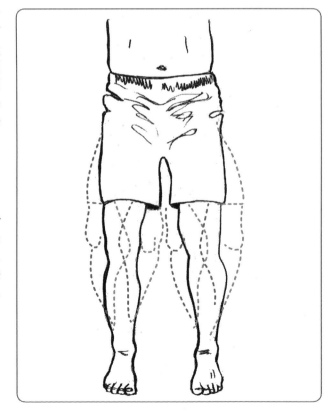

Figure 162

Hip Ups/Hip Downs

Start this exercise by standing and placing your right foot on a stair or stool. Make sure your leg is straight under your pelvis. To do this, you must hold on to something. Now raise and lower your left pelvis. Your left leg should raise and lower with your pelvis. Make sure your pelvis is dropping straight and not rotating forward or backward. See Figures 163, 164, and 165. Repeat 4–12 times on each leg. This exercise will improve your hip flexor flexibility.

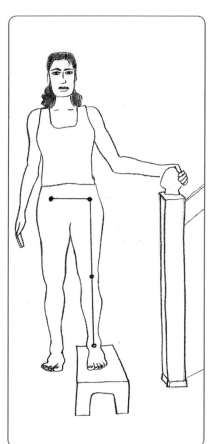 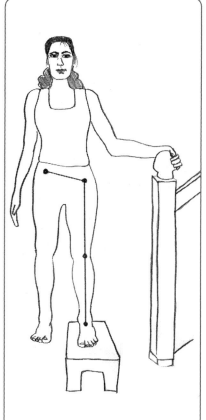 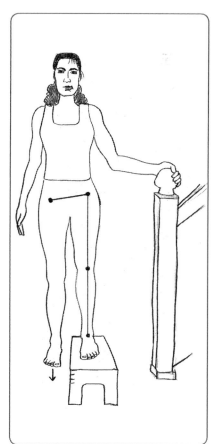

Left, Figure 163   Middle, Figure 164   Right, Figure 165

Pelvic Figure Eights

Stand in a room with your back to a wall, and with walls to your right and left to be used as reference points. Place your feet 3–6 inches more than hip-distance apart. A good position to start would be your stance position. Your knees are bent and your back and neck are straight. Your hands will be at your waist with palms facing the floor. Your hands are in this position as a reminder to keep your pelvis level. Your feet will remain flat on the floor throughout the exercise and your knees will bend various amounts to keep your pelvis level. See Figure 166.

You will be mapping a figure eight with your pelvis. Start by facing forward. Begin moving your pelvis right along the pattern of the eight. As you start to shift your weight over your right leg, maximally rotate your pelvis until it faces the wall to your right. Do this by rotating your pelvis in a circle over your right leg. Next, begin moving your pelvis backward to the left. As your pelvis approaches the center of the figure eight, rotate back to neutral. You will again be facing forward or close to it. Then begin moving your pelvis left along the pattern of the eight. As you start to shift your weight over your left leg, maximally rotate your pelvis until it faces the wall to your left. Do this by rotating your pelvis in a circle over your left leg. Return back to the center of the eight. Continue the figure eights by flowing from right to left for 4–12 repetitions. Begin with larger eights for the first set, progressing to smaller eights for the last. This exercise can also be done in reverse. See Figures 167, 168, 169, 170, 171, 172, and 173.

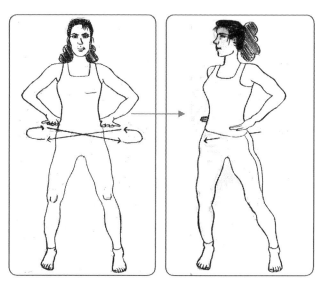

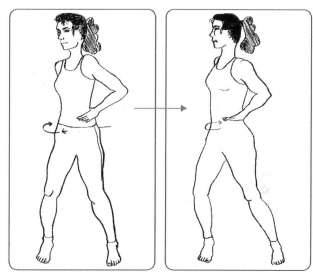

Left, Figure 166   Right, Figure 167   Left, Figure 168   Right, Figure 169

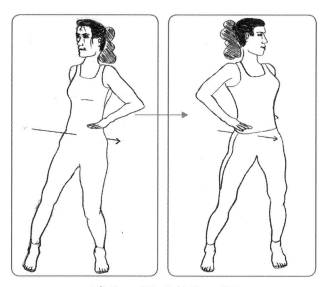

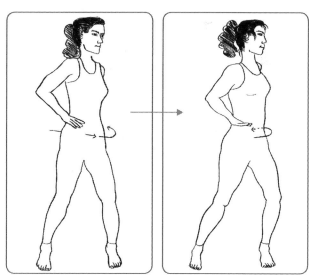

Left, Figure 170   Right, Figure 171   Left, Figure 172   Right, Figure 173

Chapter 7: Super Seven Warm-Up Exercises

Trunk Rotation

Sit up straight in a chair with your legs crossed at the knees. See Figure 174. Rotate your trunk and head to the right. Remain upright as you rotate. Place your left arm on the right side of your legs. Push your left arm into your knees, to further your rotation. See Figure 175. Allow your right arm to rotate stretched out straight behind you. Rotate until you feel slight resistance in the trunk area. Take a deep breath, holding for a few seconds and then letting it out. Repeat breathing 4–12 repetitions. Then repeat, rotating left and taking 4–12 breaths. See Figures 176 and 177.

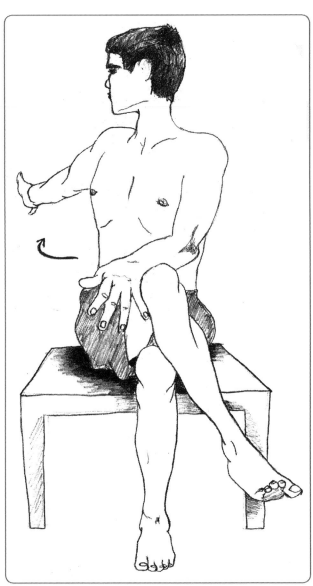

Figure 175

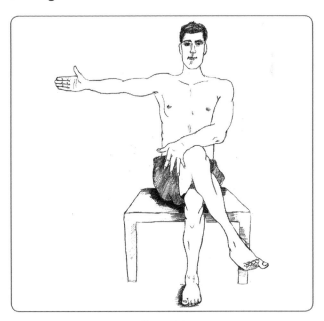

Figure 174

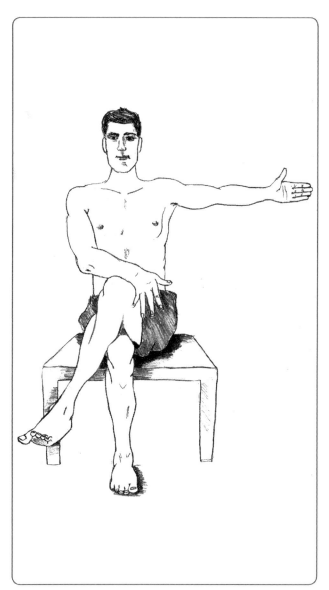

Figure 176

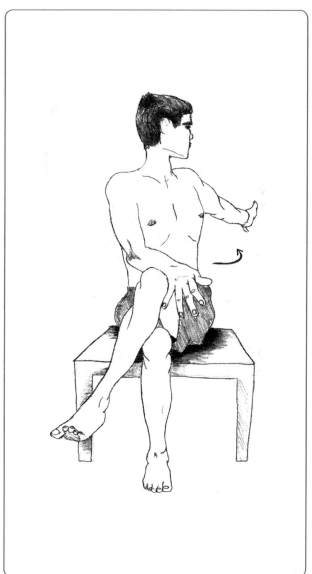

Figure 177

Trunk Side-Bending

Sit up straight with your feet flat. Drop your right shoulder down as low as it will go. Raise your left shoulder up as high as it will go. See Figure 178. Let your head bend to the right side. Take a deep breath, holding for a few seconds and then letting it out. Repeat breathing 10 times. Then drop your left shoulder down as low as it will go. See Figure 179. Raise your right shoulder up as high as it will go. Let your head bend to the left side. Take a deep breath, holding for a few seconds and then letting it out. Repeat breathing 4–12 times. Then side-bend left and take 4–12 breaths.

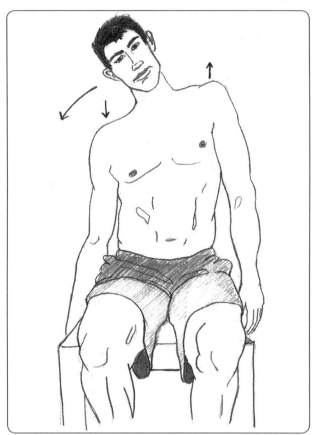

Figure 178

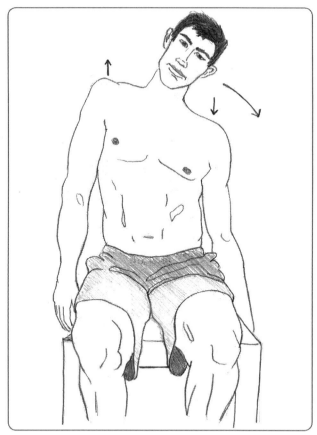

Figure 179

Modification of Upper Rib cage Lengthening (Done in Sitting)

Sit in a comfortable chair with your arms at your side and your hands clasped together. Your elbows will be bent at a 90-degree angle. Flatten your back to the chair and pull your lower ribs together, engaging the abdominals and low back musculature. You may keep your back slightly arched if that is more comfortable. Be careful not to lock the lower rib cage down so tightly that you cannot rotate properly through this area. Raise your arms over your head, keeping your elbows at a 90-degree angle while breathing into your upper ribs and sternum. Do 4–12 repetitions. See Figures 180 and 181.

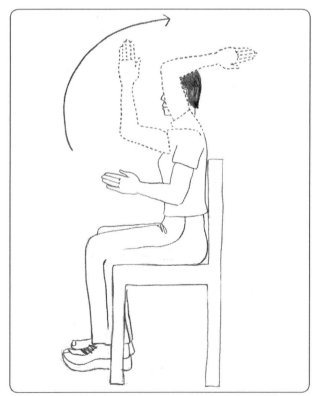

Figure 180

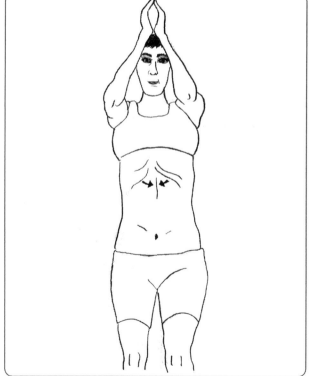

Figure 181

Prayer Position

Start by sitting, placing your hands palm-to-palm behind your back in a reverse prayer position. See Figures 182, and 183. Now roll your hands in toward your spine until they are in a prayer position behind your back. Your hands may separate to accomplish this. Move praying hands up your back. See Figure 184. Repeat 4–12 times.

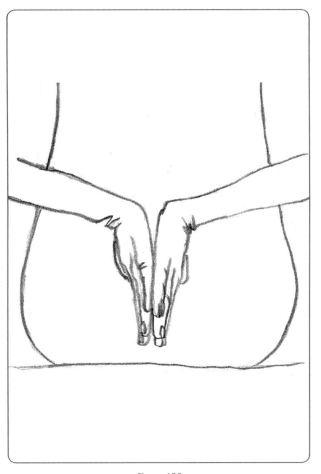

Figure 182

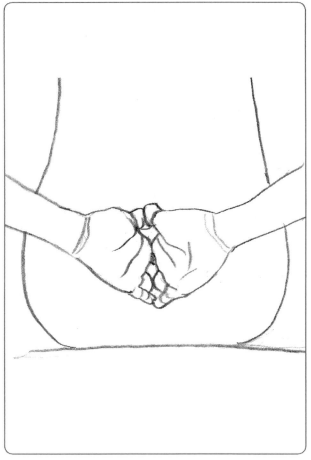

Figure 183

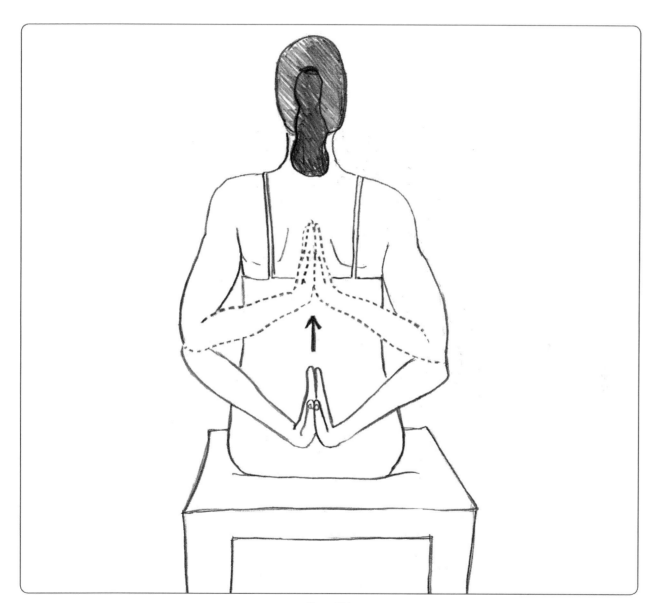

Figure 184

Eye dominance is incredibly important for a golfer and can tremendously impact your swing. For most people, the dominant eye is on the same side as their dominant hand. Most people are right-eye and right-hand dominant. For a select few, their dominance is on opposite sides, meaning right-hand and left-eye dominance or left-hand and right-eye dominance. This is called cross dominance.

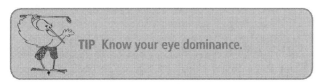

TIP Know your eye dominance.

To check your eye dominance, remove from the book the two pieces of paper from Appendix C. Take the paper with the numbers and characters on it, and place it on the floor in front of your feet. Put a golf ball on the center of the page where it is marked with the word "Ball." Next, take the piece of paper with the small circle in the center and punch a hole where the circle is. Hold the paper in front of

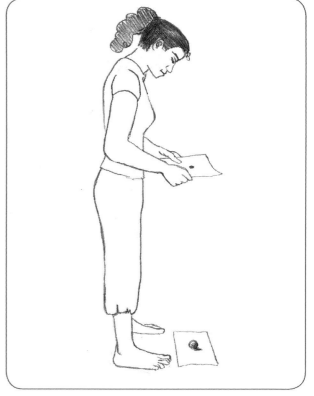

Figure 185

you with elbows bent. See Figure 185. Keep the paper in this same place for the duration of the test. Now find the ball through the small hole with both eyes open and looking at the ball. Then close your right eye. Note whether you see the ball or a character on the paper with your left eye. Then close your left eye and open your right. Note whether you see the ball or a character on the paper with your right eye. The dominant eye is the one seeing the ball.

Also note from the test how far from the ball your nondominant eye sees. This is critical because if you take your dominant eye off the ball during the backswing, your brain now has you swinging for a different spot. It is likely that many people who are right-hand and right-eye dominant have to close their eyes at some point during the swing between the backswing and impact, or not look at the ball.

 TIP Keep both eyes on the ball at all times during your swing.

Vision alone could distinguish an average golfer from a great one. In the book *20/20 Is Not Enough: The New World of Vision*, authors Seiderman and Marcus differentiate between sight, vision, and binocular vision.

Sight represents the mechanics of the eyeball and where light, after being focused by the lens, falls in reference to the retina. This is called refraction. Think of the retina as your movie screen. Optimally, the light is focused on the retina, or your movie screen. Traditional glasses correct errors of refraction, or when the light focuses in front of or behind your movie screen. The glasses help focus the light back onto your movie screen.

Vision refers to the brain's interpretation of the eyes' messages. Seiderman and Marcus define binocular vision as "the product of the two eyes working together." This complex process allows for depth perception, or the ability to see in three dimensions. Depth perception gives you the ability to see the peaks and valleys on the putting green and aim directly for the ball while swinging.

Other visual abilities that are helpful to the golfer are peripheral vision and visual pursuit. Peripheral vision is the ability to see to the side while looking forward. Seiderman and Marcus report that "a person with normal peripheral vision has a visual field of about 180 degrees." This is half a circle of vision. A golfer should be able to look at the ball and glance down the fairway at the same time. Seiderman and Marcus define visual pursuit, or eye tracking, "as the ability to follow an object in motion

 TIP Find a specialized optometrist to get your vision tested.

with the eyes." A golfer should see the ball from club contact to when it hits the ground on the golf course.

In his book *The Bates Method for Better Eyesight Without Glasses*, Dr. William H. Bates reports successful treatment for many types of vision problems. Many of his clients improved to better than 20/20 vision, the standard for the most commonly used eye chart. Dr. Bates's distinction between sight and vision is quite blurred. Using a retinoscope for testing, he infers that errors in the brain's interpretation (or vision) can cause errors of refraction (or sight) due to the corresponding messages sent from the brain to the eye musculature. During testing, he found that the following produced errors of refraction: unfamiliar objects, sudden exposure to strong light, rapid or sudden change of light, unexpected loud noises, mental strain, and "conditions of mental or physical discomfort such as pain, cough, fever, discomfort from heat or cold, depression, anger, or anxiety." Dr Bates reports, "The origin of any error of refraction, of a squint, or of any other functional disturbance of the eye, is simply a thought, a wrong thought, and its disappearance is as quick as the thought that relaxes." Dr. Bates further reports that "effort prolongs relaxation."

TIP To improve your vision while golfing, keep an even temperament.

TIP To improve visual abilities including visual pursuit, peripheral vision, and depth perception, pick up one of the books mentioned, or visit a specialized optometrist for vision retraining exercises.

Thank you for purchasing *Body 4 Golf*. I hope you enjoyed getting to know your body and now have a greater appreciation of how it works to help you create a fabulous golf swing. Understanding your body, how it works, and what it is capable of is your first step to injury-free golf. With this new knowledge, I expect to see golfers hit the ball farther, have more accuracy with all shots, and be able to play injury free into their golden years. I wish you well with your golf game.

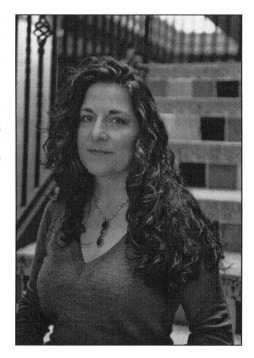

About the Author

Dawn Lipori, Licensed Physical Therapist to a variety of talented athletes, is the Founder of the Lipori Manual Physical Therapy Center in Orlando, and Developer/Author of *Body 4 Golf*.

Dawn has been immersed in the professional golf world, working with more than 100 pro golfers from every tour, including the PGA, LPGA, KLPGA, Korean PGA, Nationwide, Nike, Futures, Hooters, Senior and European Tours, in addition to the Nationally Ranked Long Driver, and Collegiate and Junior players. Her clients go beyond golf and span the world of professional sports, including pro athletes from the NBA, MLB, professional football, and water skiing.

Dawn has an extensive background in Manual Therapy and a gift for intuitive healing and sports strategy. Dawn's expertise as a "body mechanic" includes a multitude of techniques and treatment systems designed to influence body structure and organ systems, as well as focus on joint motion and tissue health. Dawn has repeatedly observed where and why golfers' bodies break down and what range of motion (ROM) is needed for the swing they desire.

"I love every aspect of what it takes to be a successful professional golfer," says Dawn. "I am incredibly enthusiastic about breaking down the body's role in the golf swing so all golfers can play injury-free for as long as they wish."

Dawn has been involved in Sports Medicine since her undergraduate work at the University of Central Florida where she completed the required courses and over 3000 hours as a student athletic trainer. She received her Masters of Science in Physical Therapy from the University of Miami, one of the top ranked PT schools in the nation. In her first year after PT school, Dawn volunteered over 1500 hours in addition to a full-time work schedule in an outpatient sports/ortho facility working with the professional men's soccer team, The Lions, and the select women's soccer team, The Calibre.

"Throughout my career," states Dawn, "I have specialized in helping athletes of all ages compete at the highest level their body is capable of attaining."

Bates, W. H., M.D. (1981). *The Bates Method for Better Eyesight Without Glasses.* New York: Henry Holt and Company.

Butler, D.S. (1994). *Mobilisation of the Nervous System.* Melbourne: Churchill Livingstone.

Hoppenfeld, S., M.D. (1976). Physical Examination of the Spine and Extremities. Norwalk: Appleton-Century-Crots.

Kendall, F. P., P.T., McCreary (1982). *Muscles Testing and Function: Third Edition.* Baltimore: Waverly Press Inc.

Magee, D.J. (1987). *Orthopedic Physical Assessment.* Philadelphia: W.B. Saunders Company.

Norkin, C., Levangie, P. (1988) *Joint Structure and Function: A Comprehensive Analysis.* Philadelphia: F. A. Davis Company.

Rex, L. H., D. O., Moran, M., L.M.P. Seminar Lecture. Evaluation and Manual Treatment of Disorders of the Cardio-Respiratory System. URSA Foundation. Edmonds, Washington. June 28-30, 1996.

Rex, L.H., D.O., Barbieri, P., P.T. Seminar Lecture. Evaluation and Treatment of the Lower Extremity. University of Nevada at Reno. May 1-3, 1998.

Rex, L.H., D.O., Cedros, L., A.T.C., P.T.A., Cole, T., P. T. et. Al. Seminar Lecture. Evaluation and Manual Treatment of Disorders of the Talus. Edmonds, Washington. July 10, 1998.

Rex, L.H., D.O., Seminar Lecture. Evaluation and Manual Treatment of the Thoracic Cage. Edmonds, Washington. October 15-17, 1999.

Rex, L.H., D.O., Cedros, L., A.T.C., P.T.A., Seminar Lecture. Adaptation of the Body to Interrnal and External Injuries. URSA Campus Edmonds, Washington. April 25-27, 1997.

Seiderman, A.S., Dr. , Marcus, S.E., Dr. (1994). *20/20 Is Not Enough: the New World of Vision.* New York: Fawcett Crest.

Whilfield, P. (1995). *The Human Body Explained: A Guide to Understanding the Incredible Living Machine.* NewYork: Henry Holt and Company.

Appendix: A – Exercise Chart

AREA	EXERCISE	DATE												
FEET/ ANKLES	THREE-WAY ANKLE													
	CALF LENGTHENING													
	PLANTAR LENGTHENING													
	FEET SITTING													
	ANKLE BALANCE BOARD													
HIPS/ PELVIS/ LOW BACK	HIP ADDUCTOR LENGTHENING													
	PIGEON POSITION													
	QUADRICEPS LENGTHENING													
	HAMSTRING LENGTHENING OPEN CHAIN													
	HAMSTRING LENGTHENING CLOSED CHAIN													
	HIP INTERNAL ROTATORS LENGTHENING OPEN CHAIN													
	HIP INTERNAL ROTATORS LENGTHENING CLOSED CHAIN													
	HIP UPS/DOWNS													
	ADVANCED HIP UPS/DOWNS													
	PELVIC FIGURE EIGHTS													
TRUNK	TRUNK ROTATION													
	TRUNK SIDEBENDING													
	STERNUM RAISES													
	UPWARD/DOWNWARD DOG													
	UPPER RIB CAGE LENGTHENING													
ARMS	QUADRICEP CIRCLES													
	BODY BRIDGES													
	PRAYER POSITION													

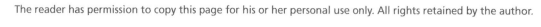

Appendix: A – Testing Chart

Name _____   Date _____

AREA	TEST #	TEST NAME	POOR	GOOD	BEST
FEET/ ANKLES	#1	ANKLE STRAIGHT			
		ANKLE RIGHT			
		ANKLE LEFT			
HIPS/ PELVIS/ LOW BACK	#2	HIP/PELVIS/LOW BACK ROTATION RIGHT			
		HIP/PELVIS/LOW BACK ROTATION LEFT			
	#3	PELVIS TILT RIGHT			
		PELVIS TILT LEFT			
TRUNK	#4	TRUNK ROTATION RIGHT			
		TRUNK ROTATION LEFT			
	#5	ARM ELEVATION RIGHT			
		ARM ELEVATION LEFT			
ARMS	#6	SHOULDER EXTERNAL ROTATION		✕	
	#7	PRAYER BEHIND BACK			

Notes _____
_____
_____
_____
_____
_____
_____
_____

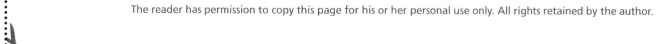

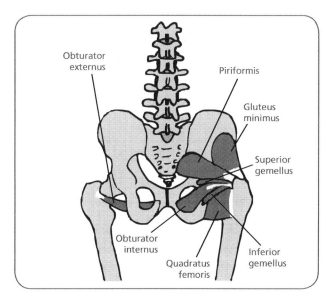

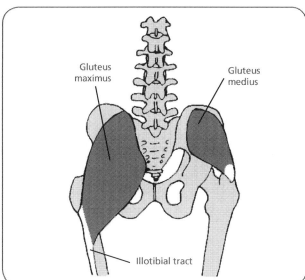

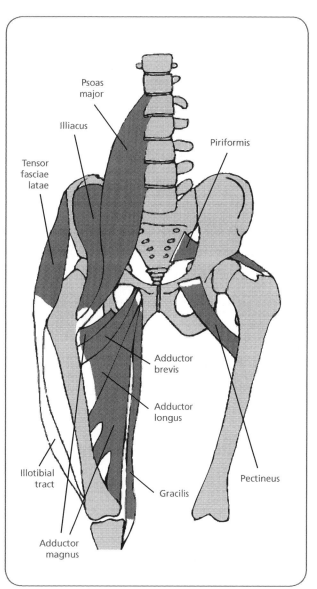

Authored by Beth Ohara taken from http://commons.wikimedia.org/wiki/Main_Page

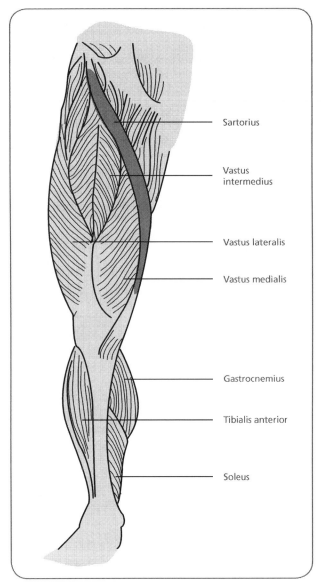

Sartorius

Vastus
intermedius

Vastus lateralis

Vastus medialis

Gastrocnemius

Tibialis anterior

Soleus

Work of the United States Federal Government, modified by Uwe Gille taken from http://commons.wikimedia.org/wiki/Main_Page

Appendix: C

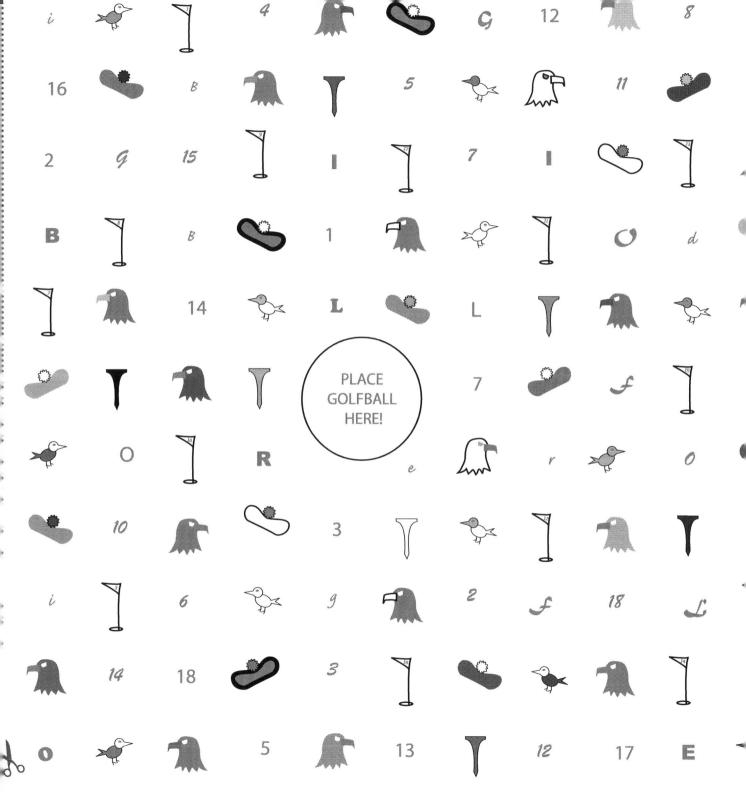

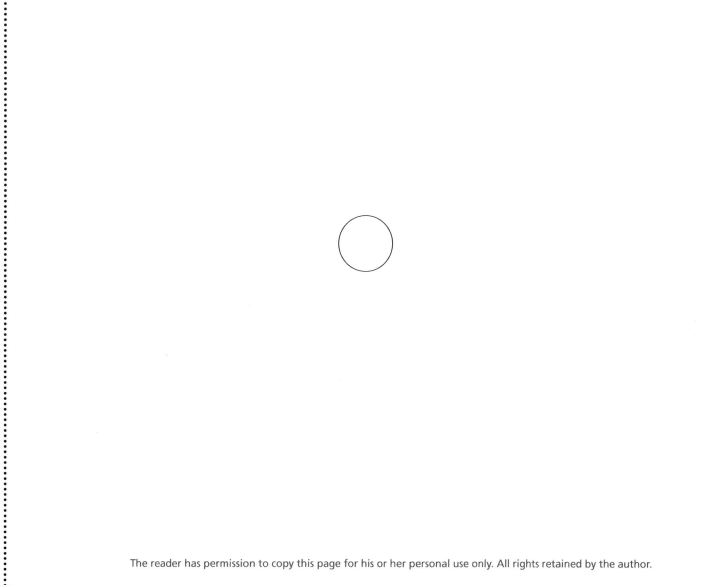

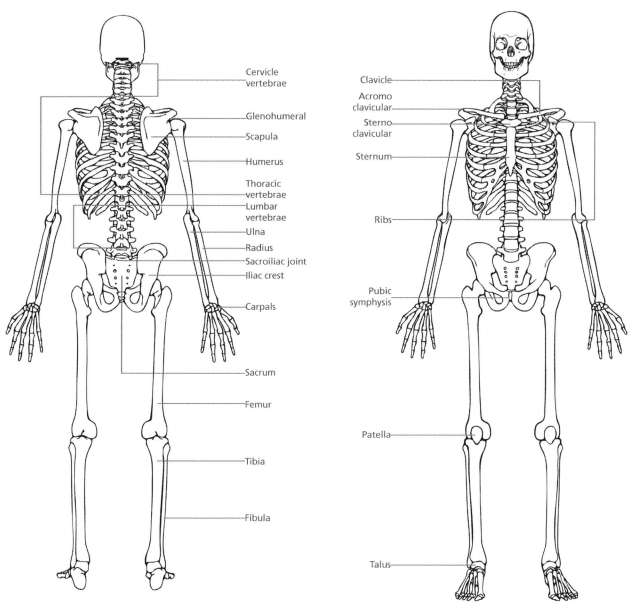

Cervicle
vertebrae

Glenohumeral

Scapula

Humerus

Thoracic
vertebrae

Lumbar
vertebrae

Ulna

Radius

Sacroiliac joint

Iliac crest

Carpals

Sacrum

Femur

Tibia

Fibula

Clavicle

Acromo
clavicular

Sterno
clavicular

Sternum

Ribs

Pubic
symphysis

Patella

Talus

Image courtesy of Pixmac/AlienCat

Index

1·11
27.95

T 563466

Made in the USA
Charleston, SC
11 January 2011